Ethical Basics for the Caring Professions

This book trains students of the caring professions, across health and social care, in the basic philosophical skills and knowledge needed to deal with the ethical aspects of their profession.

It shows why ethical education is required, and teaches the skills of reasoning that equip professionals to think critically about the theories and arguments used in ethical discussions. It demonstrates how we can be confident that we can rely on common moral ground; but it also points out how we need to recognise the influence of different world-views, and to note how, on some issues, these can lead us in starkly different directions. It explains relevant philosophical theories, and evaluates their strengths and weaknesses – particularly in relation to what is required for proper professional ethics. It shows how to employ the commonly accepted framework of four ethical principles – beneficence, non-maleficence, autonomy, and justice. These various matters are then illustrated in two extended case studies, which focus on the problem of euthanasia, and the question of screening for disability and the value of human life.

Ethical Basics for the Caring Professions is designed for use on all health and social care and human services courses on ethics and values. It will also be of interest to academics and professionals working within these fields.

Graeme McLean is an Australian who received his philosophical education from Monash University (B.A. (Hons.) and M.A.) and the University of Oxford (B.Phil. and D.Phil.). His main academic posts have been at the University of the Witwatersrand, South Africa (1990–2004), as a member of its Department of Philosophy; and at Charles Sturt University, Australia (2005–2018), as Co-ordinator of Philosophy in the School of Humanities and Social Sciences and as a Senior Research Fellow of the Centre for Applied Philosophy and Public Ethics. In these and other posts, he has been responsible for the design and delivery of various ethics courses for the caring professions. He has received numerous teaching awards, including the Vice-Chancellor's Teaching

Award at the University of the Witwatersrand (1997), the Vice-Chancellor's Award for Teaching Excellence at Charles Sturt University (2008), and an Australian Learning and Teaching Council Citation for Outstanding Contribution to Student Learning (2009). He continues with Charles Sturt University as Adjunct Research Fellow in Philosophy and as a Scholar of the Australian Centre for Christianity and Culture. His main areas of philosophical interest are epistemology, philosophy of religion, and applied ethics.

Ethical Basics for the Caring Professions

Knowledge and Skills for Thoughtful Practice

G. R. McLean

Routledge
Taylor & Francis Group
LONDON AND NEW YORK

First published 2022
by Routledge
2 Park Square, Milton Park, Abingdon, Oxon OX14 4RN

and by Routledge
605 Third Avenue, New York, NY 10158

Routledge is an imprint of the Taylor & Francis Group, an informa business

British Library Cataloguing-in-Publication Data
A catalogue record for this book is available from the British Library

Library of Congress Cataloging-in-Publication Data
Names: McLean, G. R., author.
Title: Ethical basics for the caring professions : knowledge and skills for thoughtful practice / G.R. McLean.
Description: Milton Park, Abingdon, Oxon ; New York, NY : Routledge, 2022. | Includes bibliographical references and index.
Identifiers: LCCN 2021009856 (print) | LCCN 2021009857 (ebook) | ISBN 9781032009568 (hardback) | ISBN 9781032009582 (paperback) | ISBN 9781003176541 (ebook)
Subjects: LCSH: Social service—Moral and ethical aspects. | Social workers—Professional ethics. | Human services—Moral and ethical aspects. | Human services personnel—Professional ethics.
Classification: LCC HV10.5 .M39 2022 (print) | LCC HV10.5 (ebook) | DDC 174/.9361—dc23
LC record available at https://lccn.loc.gov/2021009856
LC ebook record available at https://lccn.loc.gov/2021009857

ISBN: 978-1-032-00956-8 (hbk)
ISBN: 978-1-032-00958-2 (pbk)
ISBN: 978-1-003-17654-1 (ebk)

DOI: 10.4324/9781003176541

Typeset in Goudy
by codeMantra

In loving memory of my parents

Contents

Preface

Like many other university teachers of philosophy, I have spent a good deal of time teaching what is known as practical or applied ethics. In various parts of the world, over the last four decades or so, I have received commissions to teach ethics for courses in medicine, in other healthcare disciplines, in social work, and in similar courses for what we might call the caring professions. I have enjoyed these assignments. They provided welcome opportunities to teach students who would otherwise study no philosophy. For I have always believed that philosophy should be at the service of everyone, and that it should do what it can to help us all to think about deep and difficult questions.

The word "philosophy" comes from the Greek, where it means simply "the love of wisdom". And until recently it was the word used to refer to all learning and knowledge. (That sense of the word survives in some contexts. For instance, we still become a D.Phil. or a Ph.D. – a Doctor of Philosophy – when we attain a certain level of mastery in, say, history, or chemistry, or psychology.) But nowadays the word "philosophy" has a narrower sense in academic contexts: it refers to a specific discipline which particularly investigates very fundamental questions – questions which concern the roots of all the other disciplines. Among these are questions about how we ought to *act*, and about how we ought to *think*. Those questions are central to the study of ethics, for ethics concerns what we ought to do, and why; and how we ought to think carefully and critically *about* what we ought to do, and why. These are certainly concerns for us all. And they belong within the pursuit of wisdom.

The caring professions raise numerous questions about how we ought to act, and why. Many of these are very difficult questions, and answers given to them are often controversial. If we wish to be able to think efficiently and critically about such answers – if we wish to be able to discern what they take for granted, whether the reasoning offered in support of them is good or bad, what they imply and whether their implications cast light on their correctness or incorrectness, and so on – then we cannot do better than to learn to use the tools which academic philosophy has fashioned in order to equip us for this very task. Philosophy can certainly help us in this part of the pursuit of wisdom – the part which concerns our critical assessment of the thinking behind the different opinions voiced in answer to the difficult ethical questions. Furthermore, we may find that academic philosophers themselves offer very helpful answers to some of those difficult questions. For philosophers are not only in the business of the critical examination of others' answers to those questions: they are trying to provide the right answers themselves. And if theirs are in fact good answers, then wisdom will of course wish to embrace them.

Nevertheless, academic philosophers are not experts in wisdom. And one of the simple proofs of this is that there is deep disagreement between philosophers concerning which answers are in fact correct. The philosophers are largely agreed about the critical tools we all need to employ. But there is much disagreement about the correctness or otherwise of the substantive answers offered to the difficult questions. However, this also means that the philosophers do agree that *every* philosophical opinion ought to be subject to rigorous critical evaluation; for they know that at least some of these opinions, because they differ, must be incorrect. Academic philosophers, like the rest of us, can enjoy true insight, but also suffer lack of insight. They can make mistakes in their reasoning. Their opinions can be due to their own prejudices. They can be gripped by a distorted theory. They can be governed by their commitment to a particular world-view which leads – or misleads – their thinking. So everything they say needs to be open to critical assessment. Here philosophy needs to be at work in self-examination – displaying both its own value and its own errors and limitations.

Nor do academic philosophers hold a monopoly on the pursuit of wisdom (even an inexpert monopoly). Ordinary people, operating thoughtfully in exercising their moral sense, can offer very real insight; and the great traditions of humanity may be the custodians of deep wisdom. Or so I believe.

All of these are matters which I explore with my students. We learn how to employ important tools of critical reasoning. We apply those tools to the analysis and evaluation of moral arguments and opinions. We familiarise ourselves with the various theories offered by philosophers to guide us on moral questions, and we investigate whether those theories square with what seems to be good moral sense. We seek the philosophical insights which can genuinely assist us in finding our way through moral complexities, and, when we identify them, we practise their use in our professional fields. We note how different world-view commitments can influence moral opinion in their different directions, and we do what we can to test those influences by seeing where they lead.

The purpose of this book is to share these explorations with other students and teachers.

I do not try to work through anything like a list of the moral problems which crop up in the caring professions. That would be an unmanageable task. Rather, I concentrate on *basic* matters – on the knowledge and skills which can provide professionals with a sound basis from which to tackle the particular problems which arise in their own field. My aim is to help the professional to be equipped for thoughtful, morally sensitive practice.

I try to provide for the reader a reliable viewpoint from which to survey this whole terrain. But my views, like those of everyone else, will be disputed by some. However, if this book succeeds, I shall be helping the reader to think critically not only about what my opponents say, but also about what I say.

Acknowledgements

Much of the material in Chapter Six was first formulated in an address I gave to the Surgical Congress of the University of the Witwatersrand in Johannesburg in 2001. It appeared in the Congress proceedings as: "On Euthanasia", in M.D. Smith, D. Pantanowitz and G. J. Oettle, Eds., *Surgical Oncology: Proceedings of the 18th Biennial Congress of the Department of Surgery, University of the Witwatersrand*, June 2001, pp. 145–54. I am grateful to the organisers of the Congress for their invitation to give the address. That material was reformulated and published as "Euthanasia: A Problem for Psychiatrists", in *South African Psychiatry Review*, Vol. 7, No. 1, February 2004, pp. 10–18. I thank the Editor of the *South African Psychiatry Review* for permission to reproduce it here. A slightly revised version of that article, entitled "The Problem of Euthanasia", translated into Chinese, was published in *The Review of Practical Philosophy*, Vol. 4, November 2019, pp. 99–119. Some of the material in Chapter Seven appeared in my article "The Value of Human Life" which was published in *St Mark's Review*, No. 248, June/July 2019 (2), pp. 24–44. I thank the Editor of *St Mark's Review* for permission to use that material again here.

My work towards and my thoughts about the matters discussed in this book have been assisted in various ways by colleagues and friends over the course of numerous decades. It would be wrong of me to try to name those individuals, for I would inevitably neglect some; but I am grateful to them all. However, I do wish to name a number of friends or colleagues who have been kind enough to study a whole draft of this manuscript (in some cases more than a whole draft), and to offer their very helpful comments. For this I am enormously grateful to Bill Anscombe, Timothy Endicott, Frances Harris, Richard Higginson, Jay Hutchinson, Tony Lucas, Emma Rush, and Tom Slater.

I am gratefully conscious of the many kinds of care and assistance I have received from my family. And in particular, I owe an incalculable debt of gratitude to, and for, my parents – for their constant loving support and encouragement, and for their invaluable moral counsel and example. I dedicate this book to their memory.

Part A
Basics

1 Why ethics?

What do I mean by "the caring professions"? And what is ethics, and why do we need to concern ourselves with it?

The caring professions

I use the term "caring professions" as a rough-and-ready label to group together a number of professions whose purpose is the care of people in need. I include in that group the medical and allied medical or health professions (e.g., medicine, nursing, dentistry, pharmacy, psychology, physiotherapy, occupational therapy, audiology, speech and language therapy, radiography), social work, social welfare, and so on. I shall not try to spell out an exhaustive list of these professions; but I think we can see how those I have just referred to and other such professions are united in their purpose of providing care, each in some particular way, to people in need.

Ethics and morality

The word "ethics" can be used in slightly different ways. It can be used to mean the same thing as the word "morality". Or it can be used to refer to the *study* of morality. (This study is a particular branch of philosophy.) Both ways of using the word apply to what is going on in this book. We will be *doing* ethics as a study (we will be doing some philosophical thinking about morality). And we will be *discussing* ethics in the sense that we will be discussing morality. Morality, then, is our subject. And morality, of course, concerns what is right or wrong, good or bad.

At least, morality is concerned with this in a particular way. We talk about things being right or wrong, good or bad, in various ways; and in doing so, we

DOI: 10.4324/9781003176541-2

are not always discussing moral matters. I say, for instance, that the hammer is the *right* tool for driving in a nail, and the wooden mallet would be the *wrong* tool. I say that the Hume Highway is the *right* road to choose for the most direct route from Melbourne to Sydney, or that the Princes Highway would be a *good* route for scenic enjoyment. But these are not moral remarks. In saying such things, I am using words such as "good" and "right" and "wrong" in limited or conditional ways, or in connection with ways to achieve some particular purpose. The Hume Highway is the right road *if* you wish to travel most directly; whereas the Princes Highway is a good road *if* you wish to enjoy a more scenic route. The hammer is the right tool to use *for the particular purpose* of driving in a nail. (And if one had *different* purposes, then there would be different things to say concerning the right or good thing to do.)

But when we are discussing moral matters, we do not use those terms in merely limited or conditional ways. Morality is concerned with what is right or wrong, good or bad, *as such*. When we say that murder is wrong, and that theft is wrong, and that it is good to love one's neighbour, and so on, we are using those terms in that moral sense. We are not merely saying that, for instance, murder would be the wrong way to achieve some particular purpose, but that it would be wrong *full stop*, as it were.

And of course, the purposes for which we choose some action as right or good in the more limited, conditional way are themselves purposes which might be *further* evaluated unconditionally. We can go on to ask whether they are *morally* right or good. Using the hammer would be the right way to drive in the nail, but would it be the *morally* right thing to do? That will depend on my further purpose in using the nail. Do I wish to build a wall, or pierce someone's skull? Travelling up the Hume Highway would be the right way to drive most directly to Sydney, but I would be acting morally wrongly if I were heading there in order to commit a murder. Taking the Princes Highway would be a morally good thing to do if my purpose were to provide an enjoyable outing for residents of an old-age home, but morally wrong if I were trying to avoid being at my own home where I was needed to help in the care of my sick child. And so on.

In discussing moral matters, we in fact have a wider range of terms at our disposal than merely "right" and "wrong" and "good" and "bad". We can talk about our moral *duties* and *responsibilities*. We can distinguish between what we *ought* to do and what we *ought not* to do; and we can contrast those with what we neither ought nor ought not to do, but are morally *permitted* to do. (For instance, I ought to care for my children; I ought not to commit murder; and – in appropriate circumstances – it would be morally permissible for me to take a drive up the Princes Highway.) We can refer to good or bad *situations*, or states of affairs. (The situation in which all people have the food they need is – at least in that particular respect – a good situation; the situation in which some go hungry is bad.) Our *actions* and *behaviour* can be right or wrong, good or bad; but so can our *attitudes* and *intentions* and *purposes*. (Hatred of my innocent neighbour is a bad attitude; the intention to murder him is a bad, and wrong, intention; the purpose of providing care for the sick is a good purpose.) So in discussing moral questions, we can ask what our duties or obligations are (what we ought to do and what we ought not to do), and what is morally permissible. We can ask what situations we ought to be trying to prevent or bring about, or at least what situations it would be good to prevent or bring about. We can ask what purposes we should have, or at least what purposes would be morally admirable. We can evaluate our attitudes and intentions, and indeed our personal characteristics. We can ask what *habits* of attitude and intention and consequent practice – what *traits of character* – are required if we are to be the kinds of people we should be, and if we are to be able to achieve the morally important purposes we should be aiming at; and we can, by contrast, identify morally deficient traits of character. And so on.

The purpose of this book

All those questions can be asked about our work in the caring professions, and in asking them we are discussing the ethics of these professions. In this book, I am not even going to begin to attempt to discuss *all* such questions: the number and variety of moral questions which arise across the breadth of the caring professions are so vast that it would be quite impossible to consider them all in any manageably sized book. Nor will I make any attempt to survey the enormous literature which has progressively emerged as those questions have been raised and discussed, especially over the last 50 years or so. At a number of points, I will examine contributions made – for better or worse – by some landmark texts which have particularly influenced the discussion as it unfolded. But otherwise, I shall leave further literature for the reader's own study. For my purpose in this book is not to provide anything like an overview of the whole ethical discussion in these fields. Rather, I am going to focus upon some *basic* questions – questions concerning the *foundations* of our ethical thinking in the caring professions. And because these basic questions are common to the different caring professions, we can pursue them as a common enquiry. By thinking about these basic questions we can, I believe, become better equipped to tackle all the other, less basic, questions which cannot be discussed here, and which diverge from one another as the different professions spread out in their own individual directions.

But why is this necessary?

Why do we need to study ethics?

For many of my readers, the quick answer to this question is that ethics is a compulsory component of the course you are studying, or of your continuing professional development. You can't avoid ethics if you want to be professionally qualified. But this quick answer, though correct, is entirely superficial. *Why* do the caring professions require some study in ethics? Why *should* they require it?

Professional courses impart an ever-increasing amount of specialist knowledge. Much of what is learned can be described as "know-how". The professional receives training in how to identify and distinguish various kinds of problematic states of affairs and how to respond to each one in some particular way. (We recognise such and such ailment – or social or personal problem – on the basis of the following kind of presentation…; and we treat it – deal with it – in the following way…) But the professions have increasingly come to realise that, though their courses are crammed with this kind of specialist knowledge, the trained professionals have been given much less help to think responsibly about what they *ought* to be doing and *why*. What are our duties? What ought we not to be doing? What is permissible? What are the right purposes to aim at? What attitudes should I be cultivating and what traits of character should I be trying to develop as a good professional in my field?

And this need for ethical thinking has been felt more acutely as the professions themselves have grown increasingly uncertain about the correct answers to those questions. For during recent decades, there has emerged a troubling variety of new moral problems, many of which leave ordinary professionals rather bewildered about how to conduct themselves. Some of these problems have arisen because of changing societal attitudes. (Think, for instance, of sexuality and sexual identity, or abortion and euthanasia, or the new and very different models of the family; and of the ways in which altered attitudes on those matters can have implications for professional practice.) Some of the problems have arisen because we can now do many things which would have been impossible, even unforeseeable, in the past; but of course, the fact that we *can* do them does not show that we *should* do them, or even that we should be *permitted* to do them. (Think, for instance, of contemporary reproductive technologies; or of our abilities to perform very early antenatal diagnoses of disabilities or "undesirable" characteristics; or of new means of acquiring genetic information, and of performing genetic manipulation and enhancement; or of the vast expansion of information technology and the possibilities it carries for the investigation and control of human behaviour.) And our task in dealing with these developments and problems is not made any easier by the fact that there is a host of very *different* voices telling us what we ought to do. Many of the proposed solutions to these problems are highly controversial.

So our learning how to think ethically about our profession needs to equip us not merely to reflect upon what we are ordinarily expected to do, but also to deal as well as we can with these new and difficult problems. In listening to the debates about how these problems are to be solved, we need to be able to sort out the wise from the unwise voices. We need to develop the critical ability to discern when a proposed solution is soundly based and properly morally sensitive, and when it is not. And we need to be able to do this not just for the problems we can see right now. For we need the equipment to deal with what will no doubt be a host of further developments and issues and problems which have not yet arisen, and which we perhaps can't yet even imagine, but which will face us later on. We need, in other words, to acquire the wherewithal to think and act with moral sensitivity and wisdom throughout our professional lives.

And that is no simple or easy task, which is why the various professions require some education in the matters discussed in a book like this.

Challenges to the need for ethics

Nevertheless, I know from experience that there are some people – students or professionals – who at this point will still be inclined to doubt that we need to spend time on these matters. And they may offer one or other of three particular reasons why, they feel, this kind of study in ethics is unnecessary or even pointless.

Why isn't the law enough?

The first of these three objections maintains that the study of ethics is unnecessary because in working out how to act, we are already provided with the guidance we need: we receive it from *the law*. The law tells us both what we are *required* to do and what we are required *not* to do. And, in leaving open to us the area between these requirements, it thus also shows us what we are *permitted* to do. So we do need to study the law relevant to our profession; but when we have absorbed it, our educational work is done, for we then know how we are to act. We don't need an extra subject called "ethics".

Now, it is quite true that professionals need to be familiar with the law relevant to their area of work (and this is another reason why they may well feel that their training is all too pressured and cluttered by an ever-increasing number of specialist subjects insisting on their attention). But I am afraid that the study of the relevant law is no substitute for the study of ethics, which is why each subject has its own proper place within professional training. Both ethics and the law are in the business of answering the question, "How should we act?"; but they do so in a rather different way, with different purposes in mind. And it will be helpful to think about that difference for a moment.

First, let's note that general morality and law only partially overlap with each other. Many of their requirements are the same. For instance, it would be morally wrong of me to murder you. It would also be illegal for me to murder you. It would be both immoral and illegal for me to steal from you. And so on. But not all of their requirements coincide. On the one hand, not all moral requirements are legal requirements. We can imagine a whole range of cases in which it would be morally wrong of me to tell you a lie. But though some of these are cases in which the law would take an interest (e.g., fraud, or defamation, or claims affecting a contract), many lies – even vicious lies which can have very painful consequences in our relations with one another – would not be illegal. Or again, it would be morally wrong of me to commit adultery (thereby violating my marriage, or the other person's, or both). But (at least in my jurisdiction, at this moment in history) the law would be indifferent. The moral requirements not to tell serious lies and not to commit adultery are not legal requirements.

In fact, I can live the life of a very bad man without ever breaking the law. I can enjoy enormous, wanton greed. I can take every opportunity for self-glorification, manipulating the truth and telling lies so that credit owed to others is directed towards myself. I can spread misinformation in order to promote my own selfish business interests. I can conduct myself with contempt for those less well off, and particularly for those in severe need. I can degrade our environment. I can betray my friends. I can neglect my children, leaving them without the love and support and guidance they need. I can neglect and manipulate and exploit and intimidate and deceive and betray each one of my series of wives, while secretly enjoying unbridled lust and debauchery. Contrary to my public presentations of myself, my charades and posturings, my work can lack any connection with a genuinely worthwhile purpose. Instead, I can make a great deal of money by inflaming and feeding our basest human appetites – our vanity; our greed; our lust; our desire for gossip, for rumour, for sensation, for scandal; our taking pleasure in the misfortunes of others and in the invasion of their privacy. I can be motivated by a ruthless determination to eliminate any other participants in the marketplace. I can exploit my employees, driving them hard and paying them the minimum I can get away with, knowing that they will acquiesce because they fear the loss of their job and meagre livelihood. I can defer and minimise my repayment of debt and the settling of my accounts, even if this causes great hardship to those to whom I owe the money. I can carefully arrange my financial affairs so that, despite living in luxurious affluence, I pay virtually no tax. I can ensure that if my business gambles fail, then my own personal wealth will remain intact, even if my employees and creditors are ruined. (Or perhaps I am so full of pride that I glory in regarding myself as much too noble, much too pure, to be prone to any of those faults; and with a sense of self-satisfied superiority, I look down upon the lesser beings who are guilty of such wrongs.) If I operate with care, all of this can go on entirely *within the law*. There is a very great deal of immorality with which the law is unconcerned.

But on the other hand, there are also legal requirements which are not moral requirements. Imagine this situation. I am walking home well after midnight at the end of a very late evening in the office. The street is deserted. I come to a pedestrian crossing on the main road, where there is a red light forbidding me to cross. I need to press the button to allow the signal to change so that I am permitted to cross the road. I carefully look up and down the road, and there is no sign of traffic. I could cross the road quickly and safely against the red light. I know from experience that it takes quite some time after I press the button for the light to change. I also know that during this time, while I am waiting, traffic may arrive which would then be required to stop because of the altered light. In other words, if I press the button, then I will need to suffer the inconvenience of waiting for some time and I may well inconvenience traffic which has not yet appeared. Whereas if I simply cross the road, against the red light, I will both save my own time and avoid inconvenience to others. The law requires me to press the button and wait. But would that really be *morally* required? (If the police discovered me crossing the road without waiting for the green light, I would try to explain myself. I would accept that I was disobeying the law. For the law does not make exceptions for the situation I was in – and nor should it do so, because if it did make exceptions for all such situations, it would become far too complicated. But I would point out to the police that my disobedience was not due to mere disrespect for the law; and that under these circumstances, alone in the middle of the night, I was not encouraging anyone else to disobey the law. And I would appeal to them to exercise reasonable discretion in their imposition of any penalty!)

That, you may think, is a trivial case. But there can be more serious instances of legal requirements which are not moral requirements – indeed, instances in which the law requires someone to do something morally wrong. Imagine that you are in occupied Europe under Nazi rule. A Jewish refugee, seeking to evade capture by the Gestapo, arrives secretly at your home, urgently in need of life-saving care and protection. It would be illegal for you to care for and harbour this man. You are required by the law to surrender him to the authorities, and to his death. But surely it would be morally right for you to protect and care for him, engaging in whatever deception is necessary for the purpose. Luckily, this is not the kind of challenging situation which many of us will need to face. We may well count ourselves fortunate that we do not live within a legal system governed by evil authorities. Nevertheless, there are regimes in the world today which pose similar challenges.

And there are also challenges closer to home. Think, for instance, of the very controversial topics of abortion and euthanasia. The law on these matters can vary from jurisdiction to jurisdiction. There are jurisdictions in which abortion is legally permissible under a very wide range of circumstances, and other jurisdictions in which it is legally prohibited, at least under many of those same circumstances. And there are people who claim that abortion is morally wrong (at least under most circumstances), and others who claim that it is morally permissible. There are jurisdictions in which euthanasia is legally available, and others in which it is prohibited; while there are people who claim that it is morally permissible and ought to be available, and others who claim that it is morally wrong. It follows immediately, of course, that whoever is right and whoever is wrong on the morality of these matters, there are *some* jurisdictions, somewhere, whose legal requirements clash with the requirements of morality. (If the anti-abortion party is right about the morality of abortion, then those jurisdictions in which abortion is legal are providing legal permission for what is morally impermissible; whereas if the pro-abortion party is right, then those jurisdictions in which it is illegal are prohibiting something that is morally permissible and ought to be allowed. If the pro-euthanasia party is right, then those jurisdictions in which euthanasia is prohibited are forbidding something morally permissible which ought to be allowed; whereas if the anti-euthanasia party is right, then those jurisdictions which allow it are permitting something morally impermissible.) And so it also follows immediately that we cannot find out what is morally required simply by looking at what the law says. For the law itself – whether in our own jurisdiction or some other – cannot tell us whether it arises in one of the jurisdictions in which legal requirements clash with morality. To answer *that* question, we need to identify the moral requirements and then *compare them* with the requirements stated by the law. And we cannot do this unless we can work out the moral requirements quite independently of ascertaining what the law says. (I cannot mark the child's arithmetic test simply by looking at his or her answers. I need to know the correct answers, and then compare them with the child's answers.) In other words, to tell whether legal requirements coincide or clash with moral requirements, we need to do some ethics.

We can understand why morality and the law do not entirely overlap with one another. Morality concerns how we should conduct ourselves, in the widest and most important respects. But the purpose of the law is narrower. It is concerned with my conduct *to the extent* that it is of particular social or public significance. There are questions concerning my intentions and attitudes and private behaviour in which the wider public has no proper interest, and with which, therefore, the law should not be concerned. And there are kinds of personal conduct which can be very serious but which could be legally regulated only at an unacceptable cost. For instance, the subtle ways in which I cleverly deceive someone to whom I am intimately connected can have very serious consequences for our relationship and do long-term harm; but the police and the courts may be able to investigate and regulate such matters, if at all, only by damaging intrusions into our personal lives. The legal cure may be worse than the moral disease. We shudder at the thought of what we call a police state precisely because it is a society in which the legal authorities play an improperly large and oppressive role in the ordinary lives of citizens – a role, furthermore, in which those authorities are especially susceptible to corruption.

And so we recognise that the requirements of morality and those of law do not altogether coincide. But this means not only that we cannot simply look to the law to see the requirements of morality, but also that we need to ask what the requirements of the law *ought* to be. Take abortion, for instance. Is it immoral, under this or that circumstance, or not? If it is not, is there any reason why the law should not allow it? But if it is immoral, is it the sort of immorality in which the law ought to be interested, or not? Even if it is immoral, could it be the sort of matter in which the law and its officers would do more harm than good if they tried to regulate it? Would legal regulation impose too oppressive an intrusion into the intimate concerns of women? Or is the moral concern so great, is unborn life so morally significant, that legal regulation is called for? These are all questions that need to be asked, and the members of the caring professions have a vital role to play in the discussion of how the questions are to be answered. But of course, we cannot answer them by asking what the law *does* say, for they are questions about what the law *should* say. They are ethical questions, which show the need for ethical thinking.

Why aren't professional ethical codes enough?

The second common objection to the study of ethics admits that we do need to get our ethics clear, and that we can't just rely on the law. But it maintains that the ethical work has been done for us. For the caring professions have already formulated their *codes of professional ethics*. So – according to this objection – we need only to familiarise ourselves with those codes; we don't need to spend further precious time on a subject called "ethics".

Now, it is true that various caring professions have issued their own codes of ethics, and that professionals need to be familiar with their codes. The codes state the values and principles to which people must subscribe if they are to be members of the profession. And it is true that the code provides important guidance for their conduct. But it is wrong to expect the code to provide professionals with all the guidance they need. One reason for this is that the professional ethical codes are typically written in very general terms. Consider, for instance, the Australian social work code of ethics, which states that "respect for persons" is one of the "core values" of social work. We can all agree with that. But what does it mean in practice? According to that code, part of what it means is that social workers recognise that "each person has a right to wellbeing, self-fulfilment and self-determination".[1] Very well; but what, in turn, does that mean in practice? How is it to be applied when, for instance, your client is a girl in her teens who insists that she be allowed to determine for herself what happens to her, and who knows what she is doing, but is engaged in real self-harm? The code does not answer that question for us. In order to answer it, we have to do some serious ethical thinking. Those words and other parts of the code can assist our thinking, but they don't do the thinking for us.

Another reason why it is wrong to rely on the professional codes for all the guidance we need is that we cannot expect these codes to be complete. Each code has been formulated at a certain point in history, and with particular ethical problems in mind – problems then apparent to members of that profession. Consider, for instance, the history of medicine's ethical codes. For many centuries, the Hippocratic Oath was appealed to as the proper expression of medical ethics. But there are many ethical problems in modern medicine which could not have been imagined by those who formulated the Oath in ancient Greece. Various modern refinements of the Oath have been formulated, and since the Second World War there has been a flowering of new codes produced by the World Medical Association. But these codes have been produced in reaction to problems not previously addressed, and perhaps not previously recognised. Among these new codes is the Declaration of Geneva, first formulated in 1948, which was motivated partly by the news of the outrageous practices of some Nazi and Japanese doctors during the war. In 1964, the Declaration of Helsinki was issued, addressing problems – which had by then become pressing – relating to research on human subjects. The Declaration of Tokyo, of 1975, addressed problems concerning the treatment of prisoners and detainees, where doctors could be associated with such practices as torture or the force-feeding of hunger strikers. Other declarations have sought to address the emerging problems concerning care of the dying. And so on. But there will be problems which have not yet been addressed by any code. We are only beginning to recognise some of the problems arising from future possibilities concerning the ending of life and the extension of life; concerning genetic information and genetic manipulation; concerning technological developments which could radically modify or "extend" the human body, or which could control human behaviour; and so on. And, just as was true for the physicians in ancient Greece, there are no doubt future problems – perhaps problems which will appear in our own lifetimes – which we cannot yet even imagine. Obviously, we cannot prepare ourselves to respond well to these problems by appealing to professional codes of ethics, for there are no applicable codes. All being well, further codes will be formulated as new problems emerge; but they will be good codes only if they are the product of responsible ethical thinking – serious thinking about what ought to be in the new codes. And we will be ready to do that thinking only if we are appropriately educated in the business of ethics.

But the question of what the codes *ought* to say is not raised only by future problems. That question is one we can ask, and *need* to ask, about the codes already formulated. Some of the recent codes have been *altered* over the years, as ethical views have changed. Again, the medical codes exemplify this. Not every national medical body accepts the declarations of the World Medical Association, and not every medical professional agrees with everything in the recent codes. Consider, once again, the problem of abortion. A few decades ago, various codes declared, in effect, that abortion is unethical (except, for instance, to save the mother's life or health). But some of those very codes have now been revised so as to remove that provision, in effect permitting abortion in a very much wider range of circumstances. However, as we saw concerning the law, there are now medical professionals who believe that the earlier position was correct, and others who believe that the recent revision is correct. So there is dispute about whether the codes are saying what they ought to say. And, as before, we obviously cannot resolve that dispute simply by looking to what the codes *do* say, for these are questions about what the codes *should* say. We need to think through the ethical problem at the heart of the dispute. And we cannot do this unless we have gathered the equipment to think ethically.

That equipment is needed not only by the leaders of our professions, but by all professionals. For as members of our profession, we are required to *subscribe* to our code. We do this *genuinely*, not as mere slaves or robots, when we make the code's principles and values *our own* – part of our own thinking and our own character. We do it *responsibly* when we understand *why* those principles and values are the right ones to accept, and why different values and principles would not be right. (And thus if we find that the code is incorrect, we take a responsible stand over and against it, and we play our part in altering it so that it becomes the kind of code that we *can* responsibly make our own.) And we subscribe to the code *effectively* when we understand how to *apply* its general values and principles into the actual detail of the many and varied sorts of situation with which we will be faced in practice. These kinds of understanding are what education in ethics seeks to develop.

So in thinking about the law and about professional ethical codes, we in fact see the need for distinct ethics education, after all.

But isn't morality relative?

But I now turn to the third common objection to the study of ethics. In my view, this is the most serious and radical objection. It claims not so much that we do not *need* to study ethics as that there is no real *point* in doing so. Many people feel that there is something pointless about studying ethics, because – they feel – we can do no better than merely air our different ethical opinions. And this view tends to arise from thoughts such as those which might be expressed in the following sorts of way:

> Morality is highly controversial. We disagree about many issues, and there doesn't seem to be much realistic prospect of reaching agreement. There are, as already noted, the deep disagreements in our own society on issues such as abortion and euthanasia. Think also of such questions as sexual diversity and sexual identity. Note how our moral attitudes are conditioned by our social connections and our political allegiances. And think of the ways in which religious people differ from non-religious people in their moral views. Their differences are fundamental, and any discussion between them just becomes a matter of different voices shouting at one another from quite separate viewpoints. And when we widen our perspective and look at the range of cultures throughout history and across the world, we see enormous divergences in moral views. Indeed, when we keep those divergences in mind, we realise that we *can't* just say that something is right, or wrong, *full stop*. We can only say that something is right or wrong *within such and such particular culture*. And though I might be able to say that something is right *for me*, that doesn't mean that it's also right *for you*, for morality is subjective. Rightness and wrongness are relative to different people, and different cultures. But this means that it's quite mistaken to suppose that there is such a thing as reaching objectively correct answers in ethics. Contrast this with other subjects. In studying science, for instance, we are enquiring into objective facts about the natural world. But there aren't any facts like that in the moral realm. There are only the different subjective opinions and attitudes. So the best that ethics can do is simply describe the different moral views that different people or cultures hold. And is there any real point in spending serious time in doing that?

There is a lot going on in that objection. We need to sort out its various claims and assumptions, and critically examine them. And we need to think carefully about the large and deeply important issues raised by the objection. But that will require a chapter of its own.

Before that, however, it will be helpful to gather some equipment to assist us in thinking carefully and critically about the kind of reasoning involved in that objection, and about other kinds of reasoning involved in the presentation of ethical views. This will be our task in the next chapter. And then we will be in a position to use that equipment when we return to consider that third objection in Chapter Three, and when we proceed to our discussions in the later chapters.

This book's point of view

But before we leave this chapter, I should perhaps say something in response to a worry that may have arisen. The expression of that third objection – claiming that morality is relative – might have prompted the reader to worry about *my* perspective in this whole subject. What is *my* point of view? What angle am I coming from as I conduct this discussion?

That is a legitimate question. Every book is written from some "point of view". Each of us writes – indeed, we say anything at all – from a particular perspective. There are things visible to us, and things invisible; things we know, and things we don't. We operate with our own purposes, beliefs, expectations, presuppositions, prejudices. And all these ways in which our perspective is conditioned can affect how we view the world, and therefore what we say about it and what we fail to say. They affect where our attention is directed, how we interpret what we see, and what implications we draw from what we see. Sometimes people lament the fact that we cannot objectively report our subject matter in the way that a camera can film the world. But this betrays a naïve misunderstanding of how much even the work of a camera is governed by its operator's beliefs and presuppositions. Why is the camera pointed in the direction in which it is pointed? Why is it turned on when it is? Why is it turned off when it is? Those questions can be answered only by referring to the operator's beliefs concerning what *matters* or is interesting, and what doesn't matter and is not interesting – beliefs about what is *important* and what is not, which govern the *purposes* with which the operator performs. And then, of course, there is a whole series of further such questions to be asked as the film is used to compose some presentation. Which parts are selected, and which are cut out? How are they arranged, in what sequence, and with what emphasis…? Again, those questions are answered by referring to the composer's purposes and presuppositions – all of which are governing what is going on well before we get to the stage where there is added any verbal report or commentary. So even the use of a camera is controlled by very particular personal factors. And of course, a subject matter as complex as ethics involves far more scope for the intrusion of these personal elements.

In writing this book, I am certainly operating with my own purposes. I am selecting the topics I believe to be important (though I do so knowing that there are many other topics that could also be fruitfully discussed, if we had the time and inclination). In various places, I am going to say what I believe to be true on those topics (though I will also often leave my own views unexpressed). But I am going to try to present what *reasons* I can offer for the views I will express, in the hope that readers can decide for themselves whether they are views which ought to be held.

But still, it might be asked: what is my *starting point*? What will I be presupposing in offering my reasons? In defending some moral view, I could offer as my reason that Mumbo Jumbo has declared that this view is correct. But for someone who does not accept Mumbo Jumbo as a moral authority, this will hardly count as a good reason. So, in offering reasons, I am going to try to offer reasons that might be accepted *by whom*? What am I taking for granted, and what do I need my readers to take for granted if they are to accept that what I offer as reasons really do count as reasons? The answer to this is that I am going to do my best to appeal to what I might call general common sense. I am going to try to offer reasons which can be recognised as good reasons by ordinary reasonable people, working with an ordinary reasonable moral sense. For I believe, and I shall argue, that ordinary people do possess some common moral sense; and that we can appeal to this as we engage in moral discussion together and size up what we hear from various commentators – including what we're told by the philosophers.

But of course, it is for the reader to be asking, at each point in the discussion, whether good reasons are in fact being presented for what I say.

Note

1 *Code of Ethics*, Australian Association of Social Workers, 2010.

2
Some basic logical tools

We saw in the last chapter that if we are to engage responsibly with the ethics of our profession, we need to do some serious thinking. We need to think about how to resolve difficult moral problems. Different voices will express their own views about how to deal with those problems, and we need to listen to each voice *critically* – to do our best to work out whether it is expressing the truth. Is the view being expressed *obviously* true? If it is not obvious, are we at least being offered *reasons* for the view? If so, *what* are those reasons? And are they *good or bad*? Are they reasons which show us that we should accept that view? And can we find reasons of our own which support or oppose the view?

Now those questions take for granted something that might be challenged. They assume that there is *truth* to be discovered – or at least searched for – in ethics. And we have already heard a challenge to this assumption in the objection mentioned at the end of the previous chapter – the objection that morality is relative or subjective. If that objection is correct, then there is no such thing as truth – at least objective or universal truth – in ethics. As I said, we will return to examine that objection in Chapter Three; and I propose that we put it aside until then. I propose that in the meantime we proceed on the basis of the *working assumption* that there is truth in ethics, and that therefore we can sensibly ask whether some or other bit of ethical thought or talk involves good reasoning or bad (reasoning that can reliably lead us to truth, or that cannot). I believe that we will find it both illuminating and fruitful to operate with that assumption, even before we return to consider it head-on in the next chapter.

In this chapter, then, we are going to gather a few basic logical tools which will help us to think critically – which will help us to see whether some view is true or false, and whether some bit of reasoning is good or bad. At the end of the last chapter, I mentioned my reliance on common sense. The tools gathered in this chapter are also part of our common sense. Or at least, when we are employing our common sense *carefully*, we can recognise these as proper, reliable tools.

DOI: 10.4324/9781003176541-3

Identifying arguments

Suppose that you are a member of my class, and I can see that you feel rather anxious about your ability to cope with logic. I seek to reassure you: "Everyone in this class can manage basic logic," I say. You look sceptical, so I try to persuade you by offering reasons for what I have said, and I do this in the following pedantic little speech:

> *Everyone in this class possesses at least an average level of intelligence. And everyone who possesses at least an average level of intelligence can manage basic logic. Therefore, everyone in this class can manage basic logic.*

What I have just done is provide an ***argument*** for what I said. (When philosophers talk of arguments, they are using the term in this sense – to refer not to verbal fights, but to the reasons given for some view.) The argument has a number of different elements. There is what I am arguing *for* – that is, the claim, or proposition, that *everyone in this class can manage basic logic*. This is the ***conclusion*** of the argument. And there are the reasons I am arguing *from*. Those reasons, in my argument above, involve two distinct claims, or propositions, and each one of those is called a ***premise***. There is a conventional way of setting out an argument – premise by premise, and distinguishing the premises from the conclusion – which is called the ***standard form*** of the argument. The standard form of that argument of mine is as follows:

> *Everyone in this class possesses at least an average level of intelligence.*
>
> *Everyone who possesses at least an average level of intelligence can manage basic logic.*
>
> ---
>
> *Everyone in this class can manage basic logic.*

Note that each premise is put on a new line. Then a line is marked, at the end of the set of premises: this line represents "therefore". The conclusion is stated last, below the line. (Once the line is in place, "therefore" does not need to be written.)

Putting that argument of mine into standard form is a very straightforward exercise, for I expressed it in virtually its standard form. (The expressed "And" becomes superfluous in the standard form, for it is not part of the content of either of the premises.) But an argument need not be expressed that way. Note the following three arguments, and consider what their standard forms are:

> *No-one who is at least ordinarily intelligent needs to be at all anxious about critical reasoning, so no-one who can be trained for a caring profession needs to be at all anxious about it, since everyone who can be trained for a caring profession is at least ordinarily intelligent.*

No-one who can be trained for a caring profession needs to be at all anxious about critical reasoning, because no-one who is at least ordinarily intelligent needs to be at all anxious about it, and everyone who can be trained for one of those professions is at least ordinarily intelligent.

Everyone who can be trained for a caring profession is at least ordinarily intelligent, and no-one who is at least ordinarily intelligent needs to be at all anxious about critical reasoning, so no-one who can be trained for one of those professions needs to be at all anxious about it.

You will be able to see that these are three different expressions of the *same* argument, and its standard form is as follows:

Everyone who can be trained for a caring profession is at least ordinarily intelligent.

No-one who is at least ordinarily intelligent needs to be at all anxious about critical reasoning.

No-one who can be trained for a caring profession needs to be at all anxious about critical reasoning.

The standard form tidies up the argument, spelling out in full what is meant within the ordinary expressions of the argument. (Terms such as "it" and "one of those professions" are replaced by what they refer to.) In each of the different expressions of the argument above, the three distinct propositions within the argument were contained within one sentence; but the standard form sets them out distinctly. (So when we are considering an argument presented in ordinary speech or writing, we need not expect to find each premise and the conclusion within a separate sentence.) The conclusion of the argument occurs at different places in those different expressed presentations. (It is in the middle of the first presentation, at the beginning of the second, and at the end of the third.) We discover the conclusion not by looking for *where* it occurs, but by looking for the words that signal the *direction of the reasoning* presented. (Words such as "therefore", "so", "hence" and "thus" can introduce the conclusion. Words such as "because", "since", "for" and "as" can introduce a premise or premises.)

So the same argument can be expressed in various different ways, and the way it is expressed may look or sound very different from its standard form. But we should be looking for its standard form. This may take some doing. Actually clarifying the argument so that its standard form can be properly stated may require considerable care. The first thing to do is to identify the conclusion. Then the distinct premises need to be sorted out. (There could be any number of premises. The example arguments given above, like many other examples, have two premises each. But there could be many more. There could be just one.) But when we have set out the standard form, we know *what the argument is*. And *until* we can do that, we will be unclear about just what is being argued and how the argument is intended to work.

When we are thinking critically about anyone's reasons for some view, our first task, then, is to set out the standard form of the argument being proposed. Having done so, we have then *identified* the argument. The next task, of course, is to *evaluate* it – to work out whether it is a good or bad argument.

Evaluating arguments

What is it for an argument to be *good*? An argument is proposed in order to show us that we should accept its conclusion. It is supposed to *support* its conclusion. Now there is plenty of room for discussion about how different kinds of argument might offer different kinds of support. Are the premises supposed to show that the conclusion is *probable*? Are they supposed to show that the conclusion is *certainly true*? And so on. But let's concentrate for the time being on the kind of argument offered with the intention of showing that we ought to accept the conclusion as definitely true. Then the argument will be a good argument if it does succeed in doing that. And in order to ascertain whether the argument does show us that we ought to accept the truth of its conclusion, we need to ask *two questions*. These are *different and quite independent* questions. But each is vital.

Is the argument valid?

The first of these two questions is often asked in this way: *Does the conclusion follow from the premises?* And when we ask this we are asking: *If the premises were true, would the conclusion then have to be true as well?*

Consider our first argument again:

> *Everyone in this class possesses at least an average level of intelligence.*
>
> *Everyone who possesses at least an average level of intelligence can manage basic logic.*
>
> ---
>
> *Everyone in this class can manage basic logic.*

We can see that the conclusion *does* follow from the premises. If those premises were true, then the conclusion would also *have to be* true. It would be *impossible* for the conclusion to be false if those premises were true. When an argument has this property – when its conclusion does follow from its premises, in the way I have just described – we call it a ***valid*** argument. And note that the word "valid" is here being used in a precise, technical sense. (The word is used in different ways in other contexts, but it has this very particular sense in the study of logic.)

We can see that this property is possessed by our second argument too:

> *Everyone who can be trained for a caring profession is at least ordinarily intelligent.*
>
> *No-one who is at least ordinarily intelligent needs to be at all anxious about critical reasoning.*
>
> ---
>
> *No-one who can be trained for a caring profession needs to be at all anxious about critical reasoning.*

This argument is also valid. If its premises were true, then its conclusion would have to be true as well. (And by the way, I am sure that its premises are true.)

But now consider the following argument:

> *Every lady is female.*
>
> *The Empress of Blandings is female.*
>
> ---
>
> *The Empress of Blandings is a lady.*

It could be that the premises and the conclusion of this argument are all true. But this does not mean that the conclusion *follows* from the premises. In fact, we can see that it does not. We can see that the premises *could* be true *without* the conclusion being true. The premises tell us that all ladies are female, but not that all females are ladies; so they do not exclude the *possibility* that the Empress of Blandings is female, but not a lady. (And in fact, let me tell you, in case you don't already know, that the Empress of Blandings is *not* a lady: she is Lord Emsworth's prize pig. You might care to check this with a little research.) So this argument is not valid – or, as we say, it is ***invalid***.

And consider another argument:

> *No-one who is particularly good at logic needs to worry about the material in this chapter. But I'm not particularly good at logic. So I'd better worry!*

(You might set that out in standard form and ascertain whether it is valid or invalid before you read what I'm about to say about it.)

The standard form of that argument is as follows:

> *No-one who is particularly good at logic needs to worry about the material in this chapter.*
>
> *I am not particularly good at logic.*
>
> ---
>
> *I need to worry about the material in this chapter.*

And the argument is invalid. The first premise says that no-one who *is* particularly good at logic needs to worry about this material; but it doesn't say anything about those who are *not* particularly good at logic. It does not say that *only* those who are particularly good at logic need not worry. It does not exclude the possibility, for instance, that those who are not particularly good at logic, but who nevertheless keep a cool head and work carefully and steadily through the material, can find that they master it perfectly well. So from those premises, it does not follow that someone who is not particularly good at logic has the slightest need to worry.

There is no more important tool in critical reasoning than the ability to tell whether an argument is valid or invalid. Let me repeat what we mean by "validity":

> An argument is ***valid*** when (and only when) it has the following property:
>
> ***If* its premises *were* true, then its conclusion would *have to be* true as well. That is, it would be *impossible* for its conclusion to be false when its premises were true.**

In testing whether an argument is valid, then, we need to ask whether there is any *possible* situation in which its premises would be true but its conclusion false. If there is *any* such possible situation, then the argument is invalid. Only if there is no such possibility – *no way* in which the premises could be true without the conclusion also being true – is the argument valid.

We can briefly note here that there are various further tools that can be used to analyse arguments and work out whether they are valid or invalid. The validity of an argument does not depend on its particular content, but on the kind of logical structure that it has. Let's look again at our first argument:

> *Everyone in this class possesses at least an average level of intelligence.*
>
> *Everyone who possesses at least an average level of intelligence can manage basic logic.*
>
> ---
>
> *Everyone in this class can manage basic logic.*

We can remove the particular content of this argument and leave just its logical structure in place. When its meaning is fully expressed, each proposition in the argument can be seen to concern some relation between kinds of thing – persons in this class, persons who possess at least an average level of intelligence, and persons who can manage basic logic. And we can substitute a symbol for each of those particular kinds – say, *C* for person in this class, *I* for person possessing at least an average level of intelligence, and *L* for person who can manage basic logic. And then we can see the structure of the argument as follows:

Every C is I.

Every I is L.

Every C is L.

This is what we call the ***logical form*** of the argument. And the point to note here is that we can see that the argument is valid just by considering its logical form. *Whatever* we substitute for C and *I* and *L* in the argument above, we get a valid argument. (You might care to try it. Substitute anything you wish for C and *I* and *L* – *but in that argument form*. You can be as playful as you like, and produce whatever improbable or flagrantly untrue or amusingly silly propositions you choose; then check for yourself that, even if the propositions you have produced are *actually* ridiculously untrue, it's still the case that *if* those premises *were* true, then the conclusion *would have to be* true as well.)

You can perform the same exercise with each of the other arguments we have considered. For example:

Every lady is female.

The Empress of Blandings is female.

The Empress of Blandings is a lady.

Its logical form can be set out as follows:

Every L is F.

e is F.

---

e is L.

(There is a convention in logic that in symbolising arguments, we use upper case letters for general terms, referring to kinds of things – hence *L* for "lady", *F* for "female", and so on; and lower case letters for individuals – hence *e* for the Empress of Blandings.) And again, we can see that, whatever *L* and *F* and *e* might stand for, any argument of that particular logical form is invalid.

So it is an argument's logical form that makes the argument valid, or invalid, as the case may be. And we can ascertain whether the argument is valid by reducing it to its logical form and then applying the test for validity. Indeed, this is generally the *surest* way to ascertain whether the argument is valid or not. For by reducing the argument to its logical form, we are concentrating on what is relevant to the question of its validity, and putting aside what is irrelevant. We may actually know something about the truth or falsity of the premises or the conclusion of the argument as it was presented to us, and this may be affecting our thoughts as we try to work out whether the argument is valid or not. But of course, this knowledge would be irrelevant to our concern about the argument's *validity*. In pursuing this question, we are not concerned with the *actual* truth or falsity of the propositions within the argument, but with *whether* the conclusion *would have to be* true *if* the premises *were* true.

You might care to practise ascertaining whether arguments are valid by constructing different logical forms of argument and applying to them the test for validity. For instance, you could construct arguments, each with two premises and a conclusion, out of the traditional forms of proposition: "Every … is …"; "No … is …"; "Some … is …"; "Some … is not …". You could use the terms A, B and C to fill those blanks, and play around with lots of different argument forms (e.g., *No A is B, No B is C, Therefore No A is C; Some A is B, No B is C, Therefore Some A is not C…*), and in each case work out whether that form is valid or invalid. You will not quickly exhaust the possibilities! And you will probably find yourself thinking about the techniques that can be employed to help you to be sure that the argument is valid or invalid, as the case may be. (Venn diagrams can be used, as can various other techniques.) It can be excellent practice – and fun! – to play around with all of this. And you will find, if you wish, plenty of material to practise upon in any basic logic textbook. However, for our purposes in this book, we do not need to immerse ourselves in all of that. The important thing for our purposes here is to know what it means to say *that* an argument is valid, and to know how to put our own minds to the question of *whether* an argument is valid. In listening critically to the reasons offered for some view (another person's or our own), we need to ask whether that view really does *follow* from the reasons given.

Are the premises true?

In introducing the question of the validity of an argument, I said that it is one of the *two* questions we must consider in order to determine whether the argument is good. I hope that the other question is now apparent. In discovering that the argument is valid, we discover that its conclusion would have to be true *if* its premises *were* true. But of course, this doesn't show us that the conclusion *is* true. However, the argument *would* show us that its conclusion is true if we *also* discovered that its premises *are* in fact true. So this is the *other question* we must ask: *Are the premises in fact true?*

There may be lots of ways in which we try to work out whether the premises of an argument are true. We might simply be able to tell that they are true, for they might be *obviously* true. Or there could, perhaps, be *further arguments* offered for those premises themselves. (This process could go on for some time! But further arguments will succeed in persuading us, of course, only if at some stage we reach premises that we do accept as true.)

Keeping the two questions separate

It is very important not to trip ourselves up by confusing the two questions. I have repeatedly said, and I stress again, that the validity or invalidity of the argument on the one hand, and the actual truth or falsity of its premises on the other, are *different and completely independent matters*. So we need to be careful not to be thinking about the actual truth of the premises when we are trying to work out whether the argument is valid, and *vice versa*. There can be valid arguments which have false premises (i.e., all or some premises that are false); there can be invalid arguments which have (all or some) true premises; in fact, there are many possible combinations. (Here is a useful exercise. Using statements which are *obviously* true or *obviously* false, invent arguments of your own, each with two premises, to provide instances of each of the following combinations: an invalid argument with (all) true premises and true conclusion; a valid argument with (all) false premises and false conclusion; an invalid argument with (all) true premises and false conclusion; a valid argument with (all) false premises and true conclusion; an invalid argument with (all) false premises and false conclusion; a valid argument with (all) true premises and true conclusion; an invalid argument with (all) false premises and true conclusion. And then – before you read any further – work out the answer to the question: what combination *can't* you invent, and why not?) The only *impossible* combination is that of a valid argument which has (all) true premises and a false conclusion. And we see why that combination is impossible when we consider what "valid" means.

Is the argument sound?

So then, in evaluating an argument, in ascertaining whether it is good or bad, there are two – different – questions that we need to ask:

Is the argument valid?

Are the premises true?

If we can see that the answer to *either* question is *No*, then we have discovered that the argument is bad, and we can discard it without further ado. (Though we may wish to keep thinking about whether the fault in the argument can be rectified in some way. And because, as we have just noted, some bad arguments have true conclusions, the discovery that the argument is bad does not show us that its conclusion is false. For all that the argument shows us, the conclusion may or may not be true.)

But if we have discovered that the answer to *each* of those two questions is *Yes*, then we have discovered that the argument is good. And thus we have discovered that its conclusion is true.

An argument that passes *both* of those tests – it is valid, and its premises are true – is called a ***sound*** argument. (Like the word "valid", "sound" is here a technical term, which has this precise sense.) So, as we think critically about any argument, our overall purpose can be stated in very simple terms: we are trying to discover whether the argument is sound.

Applying this to an example

We are going to apply all of this to some examples from the philosophical literature in applied ethics. I take as our first example an interesting argument which is relevant to an issue concerning the very foundations of all the caring professions: to what sort of thing do we have a duty of care? It is an argument considered by the New Zealand philosopher Rosalind Hursthouse in her very helpful book *Beginning Lives*.[1] In that book, Hursthouse devotes a chapter to what she calls the moral status of the foetus. It is commonly thought that the issue of abortion is largely to be decided by determining the moral significance of unborn human life. Some people may already object to this description: they may feel that if we call it unborn human life, then we are already deciding the issue against abortion. But it is a description which really ought to be uncontroversial. The embryo/foetus is human, of course, because it belongs to the human species. (It is not koala, or eucalypt.) And it is living because it is not inanimate (like a rock) or dead. Nevertheless, this description – "human life" – doesn't get us very far in deciding the moral significance of what we are describing; for the cells in my finger are also living and human, but this doesn't mean that in themselves they have any very great moral significance. So what *is* the moral status of unborn human life? (Let's follow Hursthouse in calling it the foetus, using "foetus" as a convenient shorthand term for the thing which starts as a zygote and then becomes a blastocyst and then an embryo and later a foetus.) Is the foetus the sort of thing that has the same moral status as you and I have? Should it be protected as our life should? Or is it a *mere* cluster of cells? Would it be all right to dispose of it, as it is all right to dispose of a bit of tissue? Or does it have some other status? Hursthouse considers arguments for a number of different answers to that question, and the example I want us to examine here is an argument for what she calls the conservative view – the view that the foetus has, from conception, the same moral status as an ordinary adult human being. (At least, the foetus is supposed, on this view, to be like an ordinary adult *in relevant respects*. There are, of course, morally important differences between an adult and a foetus: an adult can be responsible for doing something right or wrong, for instance, whereas a foetus cannot. The conservative view is not denying this. Rather, it maintains that the foetus is like an adult human being in the respects relevant to questions such as whether its life ought to be protected.) The argument might be expressed in such a way as this:

> Consider a baby, sometime after its birth. It clearly has the same moral significance as you and I have – the same moral status as an ordinary adult human. And now consider how the baby came to develop. We can trace its physical development all the way back to conception. But there is nowhere along that line of development where we can say that at this point it *came to possess* its moral status. There is no point where we can say that *until* that point in its development, it did not have that moral status (and it would have been morally acceptable to dispose of it or kill it); but *after* that point, it had the same moral status as you and I. We can look at every single point along the line of its development, all the way to its conception, and ask, "Is *this* the point where it comes to possess its moral status?"; and at each point we have to answer, "No, there's no reason to say that it acquires its moral status *here*." But if, as we've agreed, it has the same moral status as an adult once it is born, and if there is no point where it *came to acquire* its moral status, then it must have had that moral status from the beginning of its development. So that means that the foetus has the same moral status as an ordinary human adult from conception, and therefore the conservative view is true.

The argument looks impressive. It seems plausible, and it is remarkable in the way that it draws a dramatic, controversial conclusion from very ordinary, uncontroversial observations – observations that can be accepted by any of us, whatever our prior beliefs. But is it in fact a good argument? In order to decide this, let us employ the tools we have now gathered. We start by putting the argument in *standard form*. Once we have distilled the argument into the real content of its reasoning, the standard form might be expressed as follows:

> *A newly born infant has the same moral status as an ordinary adult human has.*
>
> *Working back along the line of the infant's (or foetus's) development, it is impossible to find a point of change that allows us to say that at this point it came to possess its moral status.*
>
> ---
>
> *The infant (foetus) possessed the same moral status as an ordinary adult human from the beginning of its development (i.e., from conception).*

And we have two tests to apply: *Is the argument valid?* and *Are its premises true?* Let's join Hursthouse in asking that *second* question first.

The *first premise* is certainly extremely plausible. It is what nearly all of us believe: we believe that killing a baby would be murder, in the same way as killing an adult would be murder. (Some people, in fact, would argue that killing a baby is *worse* than killing an adult.) Nevertheless, in Chapter Seven, we are going to hear this claim challenged: we shall hear some philosophers argue that it can be morally acceptable to kill babies. We will examine their view then; but for the time being, let us simply note that most of us would certainly accept the first premise as true.

The *second premise* also looks plausible. But many people – especially as they look ahead to the looming conclusion of the argument – will wish to resist it. Is there a good objection to the second premise? Can we in fact find a point in foetal development where a real change of moral status does occur? Hursthouse considers what she regards as the two most plausible *objections to the second premise*, and she argues that neither objection succeeds.[2] It seems to me that she is right. Let's consider each in turn.

The *first objection* is that the relevant point of moral change occurs *at birth*. For from the time of birth, but not before, there is a new, distinct, human being, separate from and independent of its mother, to whom we can relate quite independently of the way we relate to its mother. And this has great moral significance.

But does birth really make such a moral difference? Birth makes a difference to the *place* of the baby. (Of course, it also makes an enormous difference to the mother. But at the moment, we are focusing just on the question of the moral status of the foetus/baby.) From birth, the baby is now *outside* the mother's body, rather than inside. It becomes *spatially* independent of the mother, but not independent (of mother or other carers) in other ways. And how, it might be asked, is *mere physical position* supposed to make such a moral difference? (How can it be true that while it is in one position, it has the moral status which entails that it can be killed or disposed of; but when it is no longer in that position, it has a very different moral status?) Indeed, the baby's position can be due to factors which seem completely arbitrary from a moral point of view. For the moment of birth might be determined by quite accidental external circumstances. Suppose that some external accident causes a baby to be born three months premature. Then, according to the view that birth makes the moral difference, that severely premature baby now has the same moral status as you and I; whereas the baby still in the womb at nine months, despite being much more developed than the premature baby, lacks that moral status (and can be killed). It seems absurd to say that the mere accident of change of position changes moral status in this way.

And so this first objection to the second premise – the objection that birth is the point of change of moral status – seems unacceptable.

The *second objection* is that change of moral status occurs when the foetus becomes *viable*. This objection concedes that the moral status of the baby cannot depend upon when the baby is *actually* independent of the mother. Rather, what matters, according to this objection, is whether the foetus *could* survive independently of the mother. When it could, it is described as viable. Before viability, the foetus should be regarded (according to this objection) as simply part of the mother's body, for it cannot exist anywhere else; but from the time of viability, it is a potentially separate and independent individual, which could be living elsewhere. And this makes a great moral difference.

So this objection agrees that the same moral status must be possessed by the premature baby and the foetus at the same stage of development but still in the womb. Because the yet-unborn foetus *could* be living independently of the mother's body, it has the same status as the premature baby. (Though again, we should note that this possible independence would be merely spatial. No baby, premature or otherwise, is genuinely independent of its carers. Nor, for that matter, is any young child.) This view that viability is what matters concedes that moral status cannot be due to so arbitrary a consideration as whether the foetus has yet actually been repositioned – on whether it remains within or is now no longer dependent upon the mother's body. Nevertheless, as we probe what "viability" means, we see that it, too, can make moral status dependent upon arbitrary factors – factors which surely should be morally irrelevant. For "could be kept alive independently of the mother" is an incomplete definition. Could be kept alive independently *where*? And *when*? A foetus of five months' gestation which happens now to be in Melbourne could be kept alive independently of its mother because there are in Melbourne highly sophisticated neo-natal intensive care facilities. But such technological support is not available to every foetus which is at the same or even a considerably later stage of development. It is not available to a foetus which happens to be in the remote areas of Sudan. Neither was it available to a Melbourne foetus in 1950. Are we to say, then, that the foetus which happens to be in Melbourne now has a higher moral status than the one in Sudan now, or than the one in Melbourne in 1950? (And that the life of the one in Melbourne now ought to be protected, whereas the others could permissibly be, or have been, killed?) These implications seem quite unacceptable.

We might try, then, to remove the arbitrariness due to place and time by defining viability as "could be kept alive independently of the mother under the best possible medical conditions – wherever and whenever those conditions occur". The foetus in 1950 and the foetus in Sudan and the foetus now in Melbourne would thus all be judged to be viable against that universal standard. But as Hursthouse points out, the time of viability is constantly being pushed further back as medical technology advances. The point may eventually be reached when the embryo itself can be supported through the whole process of gestation by entirely artificial means, without ever being dependent upon the mother's body. But in that case, if we apply the new non-arbitrary definition of "viability", the embryo would count as viable *from fertilisation*. And then viability would no longer count as a *point of change* along the process of embryonic/foetal development. And so this objection to the second premise would completely collapse. For the objection would now be accepting that from conception, the foetus has the same moral status as you and I. But this is the conclusion of the argument it was supposed to be objecting to. The objection thus ends up by accepting the conservative view after all.

So this second objection to the second premise – the objection that viability is the point of change of moral status – also fails as an objection.

As Hursthouse says, these two objections appear to be the most plausible possible objections to the second premise of this argument for the conservative view concerning the moral status of the foetus. It seems, then, that we ought to accept the second premise.

However, we still need to consider the *validity* of the argument. It looks plausible. But appearances can be deceptive. As always, in considering the matter carefully, it helps to set out the logical form of the argument. This argument is not composed of the simple kinds of proposition we have seen in our earlier examples. But we can still capture the logical content of the premises and conclusion. The first premise – that the baby has the same moral status as an adult – is saying that something, an individual of a certain kind (let's call that individual X, and not specify it any further), has some feature or property (which we can call F). The second premise simply says that in working back along the line of X's development, we can find no point of change where X came to possess F. And the conclusion tells us that X had F from the beginning of its development. So we have the following logical form:

> *X possesses F.*
>
> *Working back along the line of X's development, it is impossible to find a point of change that allows us to say that at this point it came to possess F.*
>
> ---
>
> *X possessed F from the beginning of its development.*

And now we can ask about that logical form's validity. Is there any way in which those premises could be true without the conclusion being true? Is there anything which we could substitute for X and F which would give us true premises, but false conclusion?

On the bookshelf close to me, there is a particular book which I acquired many years ago. As I look at it, I see that the spine of its dust-jacket is now a rather sickly green colour. But when I bought the book, the whole dust-jacket was brown (and the parts which have not been constantly exposed to the light remain brown). The colour of the spine has gradually faded to become green. So the spine now possesses the feature of being green. And if – as we think about the history of the book – we work back along the line of its development, it is impossible to find a point which would allow us to say that *at that point* it became green. Had I constantly watched the book during its entire history in my possession, would I have been able to say at any point "*Now* the spine has turned green, not having been green up until now"? No, there was no such point. So must I conclude that the spine was green when I first acquired the book? Of course not. The spine was *not* green when I first acquired the book. The premises are true, but the conclusion is false. The argument is invalid.

Hursthouse offers a number of examples which demonstrate the invalidity of the argument. There is the ancient example of a heap – say, a heap of stones. Imagine that a heap of stones is gradually piled up, starting with just one stone, and adding a single stone at a time, so that eventually there is a large heap. We now have something that has the feature of being a heap. And there was no point in its development where it came to be a heap, having not been a heap before that point. For there is no precise number of stones which makes a heap. But it was not a heap at the beginning, when the first stone was laid down. We can also add the example of a man who has gradually gone bald, having once had plenty of hair. There was no particular hair the loss of which changed him from not being bald to being bald. But he was not bald when the process began. And so on. The relevant terms for each of these examples can be plugged into the argument's logical form, above, giving us in each case an instance of the argument which has true premises and false conclusion. (Thus, for example, X equals "this man's head" and F equals "the feature of being bald", and so on.)

So this argument for the conservative view is unsound, because it is invalid.

We might ask, however, whether the argument can be repaired in some way. For it may be possible to render the argument valid by altering the premises. Indeed, it is worth noting that we can *always* repair an invalid argument: we can simply add to its premises another premise which states exactly what the conclusion says. (Imagine that, in the argument above, we merely add another premise, above the "therefore" line, which states exactly the same thing as the conclusion.) If we did this, the argument would certainly meet our definition of validity: it would be *impossible* for the conclusion to be false if the premises were true. But of course, this way of rendering the argument valid would hardly be a persuasive move in any situation in which we are interested in the argument because we are looking for reasons to accept the conclusion. Indeed, it would be an especially flagrant case of ***begging the question***. "Begging the question" is the name of a particular and serious kind of fallacy in reasoning. It refers to a case in which we take for granted what we are supposed to be providing reason to accept – a case where one "assumes the matter in dispute", as the *Oxford English Dictionary* puts it. Suppose, for instance, that you are seeking information about a prospective employee, and you ask me what I know about him. I tell you that he is honest. You ask me how I know that he is honest, and I reply, "He told me that he's honest." Obviously, this is flawed reasoning on my part. His telling me that he is honest does not give me a reason to believe that he is honest unless I already believe that what he tells me is truthful – that is, unless I already believe that he is honest. So in offering the fact that he has told me that he is honest as a reason for believing that he is honest, I am taking for granted that he is honest: I am already taking for granted what I am supposed to be providing a *reason for*. I am begging the question. There can be much subtler instances of this fallacy, and so it is a fallacy which we often commit unwittingly. (I need to take a moment here to point out that the term "begging the question" is now misused by many people who do not know what it means. Ignorant reporters and commentators in our various mass media, and others, now often use the term simply to mean something like "raising the question". They mention some point, and then, to introduce a further related question, they say, "This begs the question whether (or how, or …)…" (For instance: "The government is now committed to a budget deficit. This begs the question of how long it will take for the nation to repay its debt.") Their use of the term has nothing to do with the fallacy to which the term properly refers. It is an ignorant misuse of the term; and it is especially unfortunate, for if it becomes common usage then we will lose a label which allows us to refer precisely to a particular fallacy which deserves to be clearly identified. It would be like losing the name for a particular dangerous disease: we would no longer have the tag which allows us to pick it out so that we can put it right.)

But could the invalidity of the argument for the conservative view be repaired by the addition of some premise which does not beg the question? What is it about being green and being a heap and being bald which makes them able to give us instances of the argument which have true premises and false conclusion? The terms "green" and "heap" and "bald" are all *vague* terms. They describe features which do not have precise boundaries. They are features which can be acquired gradually, and in such a way that there is no precise point where something comes to possess that feature. (There are no precise points on the colour spectrum which define the boundaries of green.) Something can be *more or less* green, *more or less* of a heap, and so on. And because these features can be acquired gradually, something can possess such a feature at some time, without having possessed it at some earlier time, even though there was no *point* of time in the interim when it *came* to possess it. But now, suppose that it could be true that the moral status possessed by you and me is *not* a feature like that. Suppose that something cannot *more or less* possess that moral status. It is not a matter of degree. It is a feature which something either possesses or does not: it's all or nothing. If this were true, then it would be a feature which could not be acquired gradually: at each point in its history, something would either possess that status or it would not. And now suppose that we add this as a third premise to the argument for the conservative view:

> *A newly born infant has the same moral status as an ordinary adult human has.*
>
> *Working back along the line of the infant's (or foetus's) development, it is impossible to find a point of change that allows us to say that at this point it came to possess its moral status.*
>
> *The same moral status as is possessed by an ordinary adult human is not something that can be possessed as a matter of degree: it is either completely possessed, or not possessed at all.*
>
> ---
>
> *The infant (foetus) possessed the same moral status as an ordinary adult human from the beginning of its development (i.e., from conception).*

And now, I think, we do have a valid argument. If the infant *has* this feature, and if the feature is *not* one which can be acquired gradually, then at each point along the line of its development the infant must either have completely possessed the feature or not possessed it at all. And if there is no point along the line of its development where it *did* come to possess the feature, not having had it before that point, then it must have had the feature from the beginning of its development. So we have managed to repair the argument, rendering it valid after all.

But in doing this, we obviously raise a new question. (We do not *beg* the question! We raise a *further* question.) *Is that new third premise true?* Why should we believe it? What reason is there to think that moral status is like that? The foetus's physical development is gradual; why can't its moral status develop gradually too? Indeed, lots of people believe that the foetus *does* gradually attain a higher moral status: they believe that killing a later-stage foetus is much more morally serious than disposing of an embryo. What reason can be given for saying that what they believe can't be correct? After all, we typically believe that there are different things possessing different levels of moral significance. We typically believe that a human has a higher moral status than a wombat, which has a higher moral status than a mosquito, and so on. And thus we think that there are in fact degrees of moral status. So why couldn't it be true that the human foetus moves through these different degrees during its own development…? Those are all pressing questions which would need to be answered by anyone who seeks to convince us that the new third premise is true. Perhaps they can be answered, but it would take some doing. That new premise is certainly not one to which we can merely help ourselves. I shall here leave those questions hanging, and simply note that the attempt to rescue the argument by adding that third premise will be quite unconvincing to many people. And without that third premise, the argument for the conservative view is clearly unsound, because it is invalid.

But let's be careful about how much we conclude from this. What does the unsoundness of the argument show us about the truth or otherwise of the conservative view concerning the moral status of the foetus? The answer is: *nothing!* Unsound arguments (and in particular invalid arguments) can have true conclusions, as we have noted. So the fact that the argument is invalid shows us nothing about whether its conclusion is in fact true, or false. For all we have seen so far, the conservative view may be perfectly true. We have only seen that *this* particular argument for that view is a bad argument. There may perhaps be better arguments for the view. But the proponent of the view needs to go back to the drawing board.

Particular kinds of arguments with conditional premises

I want us now to look at a further aspect of critical reasoning. In order to introduce it, let us think a bit more about what we were doing when we examined the objections to the second premise of that argument for the conservative view, above. We heard two objections – the claims that birth and viability, respectively, were points at which the moral status of the foetus changed. In each case the proponent of the objection would wish to draw attention to an *implication* of the objection – namely, that if birth (or viability) is the point of moral change, then before that point abortion is morally permissible. And the objector is claiming that birth (or viability) *is* such a point, and that we should accept, therefore, that abortion is permissible before then. However, we also saw reason to reject each objection. And we did this by noting some *further implications* of the objections: if birth (or viability) is the point of moral change, then the moral status of the foetus is dependent upon merely arbitrary and accidental circumstances. We noted that those further implications are *unacceptable*: moral status cannot depend on such merely arbitrary and accidental circumstances. And this gave us good reason to reject the objections as unacceptable: birth (or viability) cannot be such a point of moral change. We have just heard, in the last few sentences, a couple of valid arguments, and each one is a bit of reasoning of an important kind. In the first argument, it was pointed out that a certain view (that birth – or viability – is the point of moral change) has a certain implication (that abortion before that point is permissible), and it was claimed that this view is true, and therefore that what it implies is also true. In the second case, it was pointed out that the same view has certain other implications (that moral status would depend on merely arbitrary and accidental circumstances), and it was noted that those implications are unacceptable, and therefore that the view is also unacceptable. Now arguments of these two kinds play very important roles in our critical reasoning, and we need to be familiar with them. We also need to be able to distinguish them from some arguments which sound very similar, but can lead us badly astray. It will be helpful to look at some simple examples.

Imagine that you're inside for a lecture, and you're trying to work out whether to arrange to meet a friend for lunch outside on the grass after the lecture. You can't at the moment see outside and you're worried that it might have been raining, for in that case the grass would be wet. And someone comes in from outside and informs you that it has just been raining. You draw the sad conclusion that the grass is wet. Your reasoning can be set out as follows:

If it's been raining outside then the grass is wet.

It's been raining outside.

The grass is wet.

Your argument is valid. And it is useful to analyse its logical structure. The first premise is a complex proposition. It has the structure ***If... then....*** And *other propositions* occur within that complex structure, in those spaces I have just marked with dots. In our example above, those other propositions are *It's been raining outside* and *The grass is wet.* We can remove the particular content from those other propositions, and just leave them labelled as propositions which we don't further specify, using the labels *p* (for the first proposition), *q* for the next one (and so on, if there happen to be further propositions to be labelled). Then we can state the logical form of this complex proposition as follows:

If p then q

Any proposition of this form is called a ***conditional*** proposition. And we have names for the two simpler propositions within it. The proposition which comes before the "then", *p*, is called the ***antecedent***. And the proposition which follows the "then", *q*, is called the ***consequent***.

But now we have in fact provided labels for each of the premises and the conclusion of our argument above, so we can set out its whole logical form as follows:

If p then q

p

---

q

And we can see, once again just by looking at its logical form, that it is *valid*. Any argument of that form is valid. If its premises were true then its conclusion would have to be true too – whatever the propositions *p* and *q* may be. Because it is an important and very common form of argument, it has a name: ***modus ponens***. (It is a Latin name because Latin was the universal language of scholarship when, in ancient and mediaeval times, this and many other forms of argument were named and analysed and categorised.)

But now imagine that you go outside to see for yourself whether the grass is wet. You still know that if it has been raining then the grass will be wet. But you look, and observe, to your relief, that the grass is not wet. And you conclude that it has not been raining. You have just reasoned as follows:

If it's been raining outside then the grass is wet.

The grass is not wet.

It has not been raining outside.

This argument has the same first premise as in the previous argument. And it is a simple matter to set out its different logical form:

If p then q

Not q

Not p

("Not…" stands for "It is not the case that…") And again, we can see from that logical form that it is *valid*. It would be impossible for those premises to be true while the conclusion is false. (Sometimes we need to stop and convince ourselves of this fact. For instance, in our example above, we might wonder whether it is really *impossible* that it has been raining. If we really have to keep all possibilities in mind, don't we have to consider the possibility that it has been raining, but someone had covered the grass with a tarpaulin, or has instantly dried off the grass with a massive drying machine, or something similar? No, that would be a mistake, for *those* particular possibilities are inconsistent with the truth of the first premise. Those situations would not be possible if the first premise *were true*, for they are situations in which it would have been raining but in which the grass would not be wet. The first premise says that if it has been raining then the grass *is* wet, and we need to consider all the possibilities in which *that is true*. And if that is true, and it is also true that the grass is not wet, then it cannot be true that it has been raining.) Like modus ponens, this is a very important form of argument, and it too has a name: ***modus tollens***.

But now imagine once again that you're still inside. You know that if it's been raining outside then the grass is wet, and you're concerned about whether the grass is wet. But someone comes in and informs you that it has not been raining. And you happily conclude that the grass is not wet. Have you reasoned well? Let's look at the standard form of your argument:

If it's been raining outside then the grass is wet.

It has not been raining outside.

The grass is not wet.

That argument is in fact a bad argument. It is *invalid*. For it is possible for the conclusion to be false even though those premises are true. Perhaps it's true that it has not been raining; and it's true that if it had been raining then the grass would be wet; but it's false that the grass is not wet, because the sprinklers have been turned on, or the local fire brigade has come along and used the grassy area for a training drill. (Remember, we need to consider *all* the *possible* situations in which the premises would be true.) And we can see the invalidity of the argument by inspecting its logical form:

If p then q

Not p

Not q

Those premises could be true without the conclusion being true. From the fact that if *p* is true then *q* is true, it does *not* follow that if *p* is false then *q* is false. For all that the premises tell us, there could be *other* situations in which *q* is true, even when *p* is not true. So it is a fallacious piece of reasoning. But it is a fallacy that we are often tempted to commit, and so it is notorious enough to have a name (this time in English). All the arguments in this series have the same first premise (the conditional *if p then q*), but the differences between the arguments begin with what happens in their second premises, and it is this which gives each form its name (including in the case of the Latin names). In the second premise of this argument, the conditional's antecedent, *p*, is denied, and so this argument form is called ***the fallacy of denying the antecedent***. And it is, of course, *invalid*.

Now, however, imagine that once again you go outside to see whether the grass is wet, while still knowing that if it has been raining then the grass will be wet. You look, and you see to your disappointment that the grass is wet. And you conclude that it has been raining. Have you reasoned well? Here is your argument:

If it's been raining outside then the grass is wet.

The grass is wet.

It's been raining outside.

In fact, this, too, is an *invalid* argument. The conclusion *could* be true, but it *need not* be. It *could* be false even though the premises are true. For – once again – rain may not be the only possible cause of the wetness of the grass. For all that the premises tell us, it is *possible* that the sprinklers have been on, or that the fire brigade has been practising, or that there is some other explanation of the wetness of the grass. And once again, we can see this general point as we inspect the logical form of the argument:

If p then q

q

---

p

It is possible for those premises to be true while the conclusion is false. The first premise tells us that if p is true then q is true. But it does not tell us that if q is true then p is true. So from the fact that q *is* true, we are not entitled to conclude that p must also be true. Perhaps it is, perhaps it's not – for all that the premises tell us. It may be not only that q is true if p *is* true, but *also* that q is true if something else, but not p, is true. So the reasoning is fallacious. But again, it is a fallacy that we are often very strongly tempted to commit. And it has a name (which perhaps you can work out for yourself using the model I explained above). It is ***the fallacy of affirming the consequent***. And it is, of course, *invalid*.

So we have identified four forms of argument, each with the same conditional first premise. Two are valid (modus ponens and modus tollens). Two are dangerous fallacies, by which we can easily be misled to unjustified conclusions. And we had already heard modus ponens and modus tollens employed in our discussion. In particular, we heard modus tollens employed as the argument form used to refute certain views about when the foetus acquires an important moral status. One of those arguments might be summarised and stated as follows:

> *If birth is the point where the foetus comes to possess a significant moral status then the moral status of the foetus can depend on the mere accident of what position it happens to be in.*
>
> *The moral status of the foetus cannot depend on the mere accident of what position it happens to be in.*
>
> ---
>
> *Birth is not the point where the foetus comes to possess a significant moral status.*

And this instance of modus tollens is one example of how it can prove to be very useful in our critical examination of the views we may need to be thinking about. For in our ethical discussions, we will often hear some moral view expressed – for example, the view that at birth, or at viability, the foetus comes to possess the same moral status as you and I possess; or the view that the foetus possesses this status from conception. It may be a controversial view, and it may be a view about which we are ourselves unsure. In thinking critically about it, we are asking whether it is correct. Should we accept it? Now perhaps some argument is proposed in support of that view (e.g., the argument we heard earlier for the conservative view concerning the moral status of the foetus). And if this argument (or any other argument with the same conclusion) turns out to be sound, then of course we are obliged to accept the view – to accept it as *true*. (For of course, a sound argument has a true conclusion.) But it may not be clear to us whether that argument (or any other argument for the view) is sound. However, there is something else that we can be usefully doing. We can be asking not only "What are the *arguments for* the view?", but also "What are the *consequences of* the view?" What does the view imply? If the view is true, what else is also true? It may be much easier to see whether the consequences of the view are true, or false, than it is to see whether the view itself is true, or false. And by examining those consequences, we may then be able to decide something about the view. Suppose that we see that the view has a number of particular consequences, and we believe that those consequences are acceptable. Would that show us that the view is true? No, it would not. To accept the view on the basis that it has acceptable consequences would be to commit the fallacy of affirming the consequent. (Other views – quite different from and contrary to the view in question – may have the same consequences.) But suppose that we see that the view has a particular consequence (perhaps only one) which we believe to be unacceptable. Would that show us that the view is false? Yes, it would. If the view really does have that consequence, and it is indeed a false consequence, then the view is indeed false. This is modus tollens at work. So our examination of the consequences of a view may well show us something about whether we should accept that view. The discovery of true consequences cannot show us that we should accept the view. But the discovery of false consequences – any false consequence – does show us that we should *reject* the view. Modus tollens can be the tool by which we can quite decisively dispose of the view as unacceptable – as false.

Examples of what consequences might show

Let's see this at work in further parts of Hursthouse's discussion of the moral status of the human foetus. One of the facts of human reproduction is that a large number of very early embryos die. About 60 per cent of them are naturally wasted, before or after implantation, often without the mother even being aware of their existence. But this is a fact which appears to cause trouble for the conservative view. For if this view is true – if it is true that from fertilisation, the foetus has the same moral status as you and I – then surely we ought to be very concerned indeed about the fact that some 60 per cent of those with our moral status are dying before they have had any proper chance at life. On the conservative view, shouldn't these deaths be thought to be on a par with a massive worldwide famine or pandemic or other natural disaster – indeed, a disaster much more severe than other disasters we are aware of (which do not wipe out 60 per cent of humans)? And shouldn't these deaths demand our urgent concerted action – action aimed at preventing as many of these deaths as possible? Yet many people feel that this natural wastage of early embryos is not something that we need to be deeply morally concerned about. And they are inclined to feel that on this matter, the conservative view is showing itself to be incorrect. What they feel here can be stated as an argument:

> *If the foetus, from fertilisation, has the same moral status as an adult has, then we should be very concerned about natural embryonic loss and make great efforts to prevent it.*
>
> *It is not the case that we should be very concerned about natural embryonic loss and make great efforts to prevent it.*
>
> ---
>
> *It is not the case that the foetus, from fertilisation, has the same moral status as an adult has.*

Let us put this argument into its logical form, and check its validity:

> *If p then q*
>
> *Not q*
>
> ---
>
> *Not p*

The argument is modus tollens, and it is of course valid. So does it indeed show that the conservative view is false (as its conclusion says)?

If the conservative view is to be defended, the soundness of this argument must be challenged. We have just seen that it is valid, so the conservative will have to challenge one or other of the two premises. He or she might challenge the second premise by accepting that the natural wastage of embryos *is* something about which we should be deeply concerned and which should move us to urgent action. But many people – including many people who are otherwise inclined to hold the conservative view – will have difficulty accepting this, for they will feel that this is in some way a *misplaced* concern. They will feel that this is a place at which we can, in a morally satisfactory way, allow nature to take its course. Can they be properly persuaded that they should change their minds? On the other hand, the conservative might challenge the first premise by seeking to explain why, on the conservative view, we need *not* be concerned about these natural deaths. But this could take some doing. It would not do, for instance, simply to point out that many of these lost embryos are genetically defective in some way, for we believe that we have moral responsibilities to save and care for children and adults who suffer some genetic disability. So either way, the conservative has some work to do. Can he or she show us that we have not here discovered a consequence which demonstrates that the conservative view is false?

But now let us compare what Hursthouse calls the extreme liberal view of the moral status of the foetus – the view that, right up until birth, the foetus has the moral status of a mere piece of tissue or any other bit of the woman's body.[3] Hursthouse points out that few people would explicitly ascribe to this view, but that it nevertheless seems to be taken for granted by those who argue that a woman is entitled to decide to have an abortion *simply because* she is entitled to choose what happens to her own body. This is an argument we often hear, in hearing the case for abortion on demand, so the extreme liberal view seems in fact to be fairly frequently presupposed. And (as well as examining an argument for the view) Hursthouse examines various consequences of the view.

We could list a large number of this view's consequences. Some of them would be regarded by many people as acceptable. For instance, this view does not face the trouble faced by the conservative view in the way it regards the natural deaths of early embryos. If the extreme liberal view is true, then we need not have moral qualms about this fact of natural wastage; and here the view agrees with what, as we have just noted, many people would accept. But does this show that the view is true? The argument that it does show this would proceed as follows:

> *If the foetus (from fertilisation) has the moral status of a mere piece of tissue, then the natural death of many early embryos is something about which we need not be morally concerned.*
>
> *The natural death of many early embryos is something about which we need not be morally concerned.*
>
> ---
>
> *The foetus (from fertilisation) has the moral status of a mere piece of tissue.*

The logical form of this argument is:

> *If p then q*
>
> *q*
>
> ---
>
> *p*

And the argument is, of course, invalid. It is an instance of the fallacy of affirming the consequent. The fact that a view has a true consequence does not show us that the view is true. The extreme liberal view has this particular consequence because it regards the wastage of the embryo as no more morally significant than the wastage of any other piece of tissue from the woman's body. But we can easily see that many other very different views could have just the same consequence. This same consequence could emerge from any view which holds that the moral status of the foetus is higher in its later developmental stages than in its earlier stages – for instance, the view that the moral status of the foetus develops gradually as it tracks the foetus's physical development, or the view that the foetus attains the same moral status as an adult by the time it is no longer properly described as an embryo. Perhaps it is a consequence which could also emerge from the view that though the embryo is not a person, it is – uniquely among all the things in the world – a potential person. So this acceptable consequence of the extreme liberal view (if indeed it is acceptable) does not support that view.

But the extreme liberal view also has consequences that would be regarded by many people as unacceptable. For if it is true that the foetus, at every stage of its development, has no more moral significance than any other part of the woman's body, then the woman can decide to dispose of it in any way, just as she might dispose of some of her hair, or fingernails, or some unwanted growth. And so long as this can be done safely, there is no moral objection to her doing so. If it is permissible to have some growth removed because it would alter one's figure, or interfere with one's career, or interfere with one's holiday plans, then it is permissible to have an abortion (at any stage during pregnancy) for the same reasons. If it is permissible to have a haircut for the sake of one's looks, then it is similarly permissible to have an abortion (at any stage). Indeed, on this view, a woman does not really require any serious reason to justify having an abortion. But many people would regard these consequences as unacceptable – indeed, as shockingly unacceptable. They would insist that the extreme liberal view is here demonstrating that it cannot account for the significance of pregnancy and the moral seriousness of any decision to abort the pregnancy – and thereby demonstrating that it is false.

Nevertheless, some of those who hold the extreme liberal view will be inclined to bite the bullet, as we say, and accept those consequences. They will insist that there ought to be abortion on demand. The woman is entitled to decide on an abortion for any reason she chooses – just because it is her body, and her right to decide what happens to it. Those who do believe this might be more disconcerted, then, by a further consequence of the extreme liberal view. Suppose that while some woman is sleeping, I slip in to her room and, without her permission, snip off a little piece of her hair. That would be a wrong thing to do. But though naughty, it would surely not be a *very grave* moral wrong. I did not hurt her, and the piece of tissue I removed can be replaced as she grows some more. But now suppose, not that I snip off some hair, but that I induce in her a miscarriage (perhaps by giving her a painless injection, and without otherwise causing harm or pain to her). On the extreme liberal view, this would be no more wrong than my removal of the piece of hair. Once again, I did not hurt her, and I have removed something which she could replace. In each case I have merely caused the removal of a replaceable piece of tissue. Yet surely I *have* done her a very grave wrong in inducing the miscarriage. And surely many of those who are inclined to hold the extreme liberal view would protest against my action as very gravely wrong. So we have an argument:

> *If the foetus (from fertilisation) has the moral status of a mere piece of tissue, then if I were to induce in a woman a (safe and painless) miscarriage, against her will, I would not do her a very grave wrong.*
>
> *It is not the case that if I were to induce in a woman a (safe and painless) miscarriage, against her will, I would not do her a very grave wrong.*
>
> ---
>
> *It is not the case that the foetus (from fertilisation) has the moral status of a mere piece of tissue.*

This is an instance of modus tollens, and is, of course, valid. Its conclusion is that the extreme liberal view is false; so is there some way in which the person who wishes to hold that view can resist the argument by challenging one of the premises? Many extreme liberals – especially those who are most inclined to stress the importance of the woman's unconstrained right to choose whether or not to have an abortion – will feel that the second premise is true. (And surely it is true: by inducing in her a miscarriage, I would surely be doing a very grave wrong – including a very grave wrong *to her*.) So can they challenge the first premise? But this premise seems merely to spell out an implication of the extreme liberal view. If the foetus has no higher moral status than any other part of the woman's body, then when I remove it, I am doing nothing more serious than when I remove some of her hair. As Hursthouse points out, the extreme liberal may well wish to respond to this by claiming that the foetus is a *special* piece of tissue, *not* just like any other part of the woman's body. But to make this claim is not only to reject the first premise; it is to abandon the extreme liberal view. And it would open the door to a whole new set of possible implications – perhaps, for example, that a special kind of wrong can be done, by the woman herself, or by a third party, in destroying this tissue, and that the father can have a special interest in what happens to it, and so on.

But if the first premise remains unaltered, the argument appears to be sound. It does seem to show that the extreme liberal view, as it stands, is unacceptable. And interestingly enough, it looks as if it is an argument which could well be persuasive to the person who inclines to the extreme liberal view – for it concentrates upon an implication which that person seems very likely to find unacceptable.

Remembering the uses and dangers and limitations of these particular kinds of arguments

In that way, then, we can use the consequences of some moral view to put the view to the test. But we need to keep in mind just how much, and how little, the consequences might show about the view. Let us review this by running through a series of questions and answers. (I invite you to work out the answer to each question before I state it in its following paragraph.)

Suppose that we know that some view is true, and we know that something is a consequence of this view. Do we have to accept this consequence?

The answer is Yes. Again, let's call the view *p* and the consequence *q*. Then, in knowing that *q* is a consequence of the view, we know that *if p then q*. And in knowing that the view is true, we know that *p*. We thereby know the truth of the premises of an argument in the form modus ponens, which is, of course, valid. So we know that the conclusion, *q*, must be true. We must accept the consequence of the view we know to be true.

Suppose that we are trying to work out whether some view is true, and we realise that we ought to accept something that is a consequence of the view. Have we shown that we ought to accept the view?

The answer is No. We have realised that q is true, while seeing that *if p then q*. But this does not entitle us to decide that p is true. To argue from those premises to that conclusion would be to commit the fallacy of affirming the consequent. For all that we have seen so far, the view could be false. (Perhaps other views have the same consequence.)

Suppose that we know that some view is false, and we realise that something is a consequence of that view. Have we shown that this consequence is unacceptable?

The answer is No. We know that p is false, while realising that *if p then q*. But this does not show us that q is false. To argue that it does would be to commit the fallacy of denying the antecedent. For all we have seen so far, q could be true. (Perhaps there is a true view which has the same consequence.)

Suppose that we are trying to work out whether some view is true, and we realise that some consequence of the view is unacceptable. Have we shown that the view is unacceptable?

The answer is Yes. We have realised that q is false, while realising that it is true that *if p then q*. We have thereby seen the truth of the premises of an argument in the form modus tollens, which is, of course, valid. So its conclusion, that p is false, must be true. We cannot accept the view.

Suppose that we accept some view. Somebody tells us that this view has an unacceptable consequence, q, and that we therefore ought to give up our view. We agree that q is unacceptable. How could we consistently argue that we do *not* have to give up our view?

We accept that p, and we accept that *not-q*. If we can see that q is indeed a consequence of p, then if we continue to accept *not-q*, we must change our minds and accept *not-p*. For we are then accepting the premises of an argument in the form modus tollens. And so we must give up our view. However, we have merely *been told* that q is a consequence of p. Perhaps it is not a consequence after all. If we can argue that it is not – if we can argue that *if p then q* is not true – then (for all that we have seen so far) we can continue to believe our view. (We would be arguing that the first premise of the modus tollens argument is in fact false.)

So we can produce a decisive test of a view when we can show that it has some false consequence. Modus tollens then allows us to see that the view is false. But otherwise the consequences of a view do not enable us to test the view. Its consequences can ***falsify*** the view, but they cannot ***verify*** it. To verify the view, we will need to find decisive arguments in its support.

Of course, this use of consequences to test a view, limited as it is, depends on our being able to make moral judgements of those consequences independently of what the view tells us. I can observe that the grass is not wet even if I have not directly observed whether it has been raining; and similarly, I can often recognise that some consequence of a view is unacceptable even if I cannot directly recognise whether the view is true. If the view gave me my only relevant moral information, then I would have no independent way to evaluate its consequences; I would simply have to accept its consequences. But, as we have seen in some of the examples above, we are often able to perform our own independent moral assessment of the view's consequences, and this is because we operate with our own moral common sense – as I described it at the end of the previous chapter. We often have our own moral intuitions concerning the view's consequences, and these intuitions may be clear enough for us to recognise that one or other consequence is unacceptable. For an ethical view to be accepted, it needs to withstand the critical scrutiny applied to it by our own independent moral sense.

I noted earlier that we can be assessing the consequences of some view as part of the process in which we are also examining the arguments for that view. But when we are pursuing this process in wrestling with a difficult ethical problem, we can easily be uncertain about how to make progress. We may be presented with what sounds like a very persuasive argument in support of the view. On the other hand, our own intuitions may produce in us moral qualms about the consequences of the view. Thus, we can find ourselves in a tension between argument and intuitions. Do we accept the argument as sound and accept the consequences of the view – suppressing and revising, if we can, our intuitions? Or do we trust the intuitions and reject the view, judging that there must be something wrong with the argument in its support? There is no simple formula to apply here. We must strive to work out where the moral truth lies. Do reason and our own moral evaluation of the premises of the argument convince us that it is genuinely sound? Or are our own intuitions clear enough and powerful enough to show us that the view's consequences really are unacceptable? We need to do our best to allow these different factors to exert their rightful force, weighing each against the other in order to find the proper resultant. Philosophers sometimes refer to this process by using the term ***reflective equilibrium*** – a term coined by the American philosopher John Rawls. By thinking about, reflecting upon, the different factors, we are trying to find the correct balance, equilibrium, between them.

Inference to the best explanation

Before we leave these forms of argument which have conditional premises, I want to address what might have been a nagging worry. Let's recall the case in which you go outside to look at the condition of the grass, knowing that if it has been raining then the grass *is* wet. You observe that the grass *is* wet, and you conclude that it has been raining. I said that this was a fallacious inference – an instance of the fallacy of affirming the consequent. But this might have been worrying you. You can agree that there are other *possible* explanations of the wetness of the grass (sprinklers and fire brigade and what not); but you might well feel that there are many situations in which rain would certainly be the most *probable* explanation – probable enough, perhaps, to entitle you to conclude that it *has* been raining. The wetness of the grass may provide adequate *evidence* that it has been raining. Perhaps the wetness of the grass doesn't *verify* that it has been raining in the strictest sense of *proving* that it's true. But surely it could provide enough support to justify us in *accepting* that it's true. So isn't it in fact misleading to say that the inference is fallacious?

You are quite right to insist that rain could be the most probable explanation, and that there are many possible situations in which you would be justified in concluding that it has been raining. But this is because you will, in those situations, have a good deal more information than simply the premise *if it's been raining then the grass is wet*. In those situations, you will realise that rain provides the *best explanation* of the wetness of the grass; and you will be able to realise this because you know *not only* that if it has been raining then the grass is very likely to be wet, *but also* that if it has *not* been raining then the grass is *not* very likely to be wet. (That, at least, is to put the gist of the matter in crude terms.) You are aware, that is to say, of a number of different likelihoods, or probabilities; and you realise that, taken together, they show that rain provides the most probable explanation of the wetness of the grass. You are aware of how likely it is that the grass will be wet if it *has* been raining. (Does the grass happen to be under the cover of an enormous overhead tarpaulin…?) You will have some sense of how likely it is that the grass will be wet if it *has not* been raining but one of the *other* possible explanations is true. (Would sprinklers cause this sort of wetness? Would the fire brigade have been likely to target the grass…?) And – very importantly – you will have a sense of the likelihood of rain, on the one hand, and of the other possible explanations, on the other, *regardless* of your observation of the wetness of the grass. (Was rain forecast this morning? Are there rain clouds visible in the right direction? Are there sprinklers in this area, and are they likely to be turned on at this time? Is the fire brigade *really* at all likely to be practising here…?) Taken together, these different likelihoods can show us *both* that the grass is *likely* to be wet if it *has* been raining *and* that it is *unlikely* to be wet if it *hasn't* been raining. Again, that is to put the matter crudely. Those different likelihoods can be gathered and the relations between them expressed more precisely, and this can show us more precisely how they determine the probability that it has been raining given that the grass is wet, and therefore how they answer the question whether rain provides the best explanation of the wetness of the grass.[4] We do not need to explore those precise details here. But we can recognise that we are operating with a working understanding of those different likelihoods when, observing the condition of the grass, we conclude that it has been raining (or at least that this is very likely). We are working, in other words, with a good deal of information. It *would* be fallacious to conclude that it's been raining on the basis merely of the premises "if it has been raining then the grass is wet" and "the grass is wet". But this is not what we are doing when we conclude that it has been raining by recognising that this provides the best explanation of the wetness of the grass. In reaching that justified conclusion, we are relying on much more information than is provided by the premises of the fallacy of affirming the consequent.

That kind of reasoning – ***inference to the best explanation*** – is very common in the empirical sciences and in our ordinary life. We observe something in the world (e.g., the wetness of grass, or the data from some sophisticated laboratory experiment), and we conclude that something that we have not observed directly (e.g., that it has been raining, or something stated by some more complex hypothesis or theory) provides the best explanation of what is observed. It is not the kind of inference commonly used in our moral reasoning. Nevertheless, we will note an interesting example of this kind of inference later in the book.

Further examples, with thought experiments

I want now to round off this chapter on logical tools by looking at some arguments in a celebrated article which has been studied by philosophers and students in these fields since it was first published in 1971 – the article "A Defense of Abortion" by the American philosopher Judith Jarvis Thomson.[5] There are a number of reasons why Thomson's article is particularly interesting and worthy of study. First, she offers a rather surprising kind of defence of abortion, for her case presumes that the human foetus is, from the moment of conception, a *person*. Now Thomson does not herself believe this. But she points out that in the wider debate about abortion, most of the argument has centred upon the question of the moral status of the foetus: opposition to abortion has typically simply relied upon the view that the foetus is an individual human being, or a person, with the right to life, and defence of abortion has typically simply relied upon the view that the foetus is a mere piece of tissue. And Thomson believes that this is a mistake. She believes, and in her article seeks to show, that abortion would be morally permissible *even if* the foetus *were* a person.

So she *presumes this* for the sake of her discussion. But for our purposes, the main reason why her article repays careful study is that she employs a number of ingenious imaginary stories in making her case, and we can learn a good deal, and add to our logical repertoire, by examining them.

Thomson introduces her case by asking how one might suppose that we can argue from the claim that the foetus is a person to the conclusion that abortion is wrong:

> Something like this, I take it. Every person has a right to life. So the fetus has a right to life. No doubt the mother has a right to decide what shall happen in and to her body; everyone would grant that. But surely a person's right to life is stronger and more stringent than the mother's right to decide what happens in and to her body, and so outweighs it. So the fetus may not be killed; an abortion may not be performed.[6]

Here, then, Thomson has presented what she takes to be the anti-abortion argument, which proceeds from the view that the foetus is a person. And she comments that this argument "sounds plausible". However, she immediately goes on to add: "But now let me ask you to imagine this." And she introduces her most famous imaginary situation:

> You wake up in the morning to find yourself back to back in bed with an unconscious violinist. A famous unconscious violinist. He has been found to have a fatal kidney ailment, and the Society of Music Lovers has canvassed all the available medical records and found that you alone have the right blood type to help. They have therefore kidnapped you, and last night the violinist's circulatory system was plugged into yours, so that your kidneys can be used to extract poisons from his blood as well as your own. The director of the hospital now tells you, "Look, we're sorry the Society of Music Lovers did this to you – we would never have permitted it if we had known. But still, they did it, and the violinist is now plugged into you. To unplug you would be to kill him. But never mind, it's only for nine months. By then he will have recovered from his ailment, and can safely be unplugged from you." Is it morally incumbent on you to accede to this situation? No doubt it would be very nice of you if you did, a great kindness. But do you *have* to accede to it? What if it were not nine months, but nine years? Or longer still? What if the director of the hospital says, "Tough luck, I agree, but you've now got to stay in bed, with the violinist plugged into you, for the rest of your life. Because remember this. All persons have a right to life, and violinists are persons. Granted you have a right to decide what happens in and to your body, but a person's right to life outweighs your right to decide what happens in and to your body. So you cannot ever be unplugged from him." I imagine that you would regard this as outrageous, which suggests that something really is wrong with that plausible-sounding argument I mentioned a moment ago.[7]

This has come to be known as Thomson's violinist case. (There is no particular reason why it concerns a violinist; but it does.) It is always interesting for a teacher to observe students' reactions to this case when they first meet it. Some students are irritated by it: they don't see how a ridiculously unrealistic situation like this should be brought into a discussion of the morally serious problem of abortion. We may well sympathise with that reaction. But it is important for us not to let it obstruct our view of what Thomson is doing in using the violinist case. She is presenting it as what we call a ***thought experiment***. In performing a thought experiment, we imagine a situation – it need only be a *conceivable* situation – which allows us to put something to the test. For Thomson's purposes, it does not matter that the situation described by her violinist case is entirely imaginary, indeed bizarre. What matters is that it allows us to *test* the anti-abortion *argument* that she introduced. For she has, with her thought experiment, imagined a situation to which the *same argument* (in its essentials) *would apply*, but here the argument would give us (she claims) a *false conclusion*. (She puts the argument into the mouth of the hospital director, and suggests that here it leads to an "outrageous" conclusion.) And this, as she says, "suggests that something really is wrong with that plausible-sounding argument". So what we need to consider is whether her thought experiment does provide a proper test of that anti-abortion argument. If Thomson is right to claim that the proponent of the argument would be bound to apply it to her imagined case, and that the argument renders a false conclusion for that case, then she is surely correct in saying that this shows that there is something wrong with the argument. (She does not at this stage of her case try to specify just what is wrong with the argument. Perhaps it is invalid. Perhaps some premise is false. But there must be something wrong with it. Later on, she seeks to pinpoint its mistake.)

All the same, we might remain dissatisfied with the violinist case because we are struck by the differences between it and pregnancy. For of course, there are many respects in which the violinist case is not analogous to pregnancy. In the violinist case, you have been kidnapped (which would make it analogous only to pregnancy due to rape). In the violinist case, you are bedridden next to a stranger for the whole of the relevant period – which, fortunately, is not the case in normal pregnancy. And there are, of course, other very significant differences. If you stay hooked up to the violinist and save his life, you and he can, at the end of the required period, kiss one another goodbye (presuming that you are still on speaking terms) and, if you choose, never see one another again. But things are by no means so simple if you go through with a pregnancy: you then have a *baby* on your hands! Nor does the violinist case capture your *special relationship* to the foetus – and child, if it is born. (The violinist is not *yours*, in the way that the foetus/child is.) Nor does the violinist case capture the involvement of the relationship with the *father*. And so on.

Now these disanalogies will certainly matter if Thomson wishes to draw from the violinist case any moral conclusion about pregnancy and abortion. But they need not matter if she uses it for her more limited purpose of performing her precise thought experiment – putting that anti-abortion argument to the test. However different the violinist case is from real pregnancy, if the premises of that anti-abortion argument do apply to the case, and do render a false conclusion in the case, then this does show that something is wrong with that argument.

But we might also worry about whether that argument *does* render a false conclusion in the violinist case. What *ought* you to do, in fact, if you wake up back to back in bed with the unconscious violinist? Let's take fully seriously the fact that if you unplug him then he dies. Whereas if you stay hooked up to him for nine months, you save his life. Thomson seems to think that you will accept that it is quite permissible to unplug yourself. But in my experience, many of us have genuine moral qualms about that conclusion. We feel that it is at least not at all *obvious* that it is perfectly acceptable to unplug ourselves. We feel that there would be *something* morally unsatisfactory about this.[8] Thomson seeks to fortify the thought experiment by adjusting the required period of time. What if it were not for nine months, but nine years, or the rest of your life? On the other hand, what if it were for only nine days, or nine hours, or nine minutes? Do considerations such as these make a difference to our moral conclusions? *Should they* make a difference? These are interesting and important moral questions. Nevertheless, I think that Thomson can still insist that she is performing a successful thought experiment even if we are not clear about what we really should do in the violinist case. For, she could say, the anti-abortion argument which she is putting to the test claims that a clear conclusion can be drawn from its premises. And if those premises do apply to the violinist case, and yet it is not clear that this conclusion would be justified in that case, then the violinist case does after all show that there is something wrong with that argument. And if there is something wrong with it, the argument needs to be discarded. (However, our thoughts about the differences between the violinist case and real pregnancy, and about just what our moral duty would be in the violinist case, might well assist us as we consider whether the argument can be repaired, and as we think more generally about the morality of abortion.)

Earlier in this chapter, we noted how to test the validity of an argument. We saw the need to ask whether any instance of that form of argument could have true premises but false conclusion. And we noted as an example a particular argument for the conservative view of the moral status of the foetus, recognising that such situations as a gradual changing of colour or of going bald or of building a heap would provide that argument with actually true premises but an actually false conclusion. In imagining those situations, we were performing a kind of thought experiment which put that argument to the test. But Thomson's kind of thought experiment has a wider applicability than that. Thomson does not need to find a possible situation in which the premises of the argument would actually be true. She need only find a situation to which the person who proposes the argument would be bound *to apply* the argument. She is challenging us to recognise that if we do accept that argument in the case of pregnancy, then we should also accept it in the violinist case, for it would apply to each situation. (And because it gives us the wrong conclusion in the violinist case, we should recognise that there is something wrong with it, and consequently not apply it to pregnancy.) For the purposes of her thought experiment, Thomson does not need to find a possible situation in which the premises of the argument would actually be true. Perhaps what is wrong with the argument is that one or other of its general premises is false. (Perhaps, for instance, the argument is mistaken in supposing that it is generally true that someone's right to life outweighs someone else's right to decide what happens in and to her body.) Thomson need only imagine a situation to which the proponent of the argument would be bound to apply the argument, but in which the argument's conclusion would be false. So we see here how a fertile imagination can in fact be a very powerful critical tool. Can we imagine situations – they need only be merely conceivable situations – which put proposed arguments to the test in just that way?

In demonstrating the unsoundness of that anti-abortion argument, what has Thomson shown us about the morality of abortion? Has she shown that abortion is permissible? The answer, of course, is No. She has shown us nothing about the morality of abortion. She has merely shown us that there is something wrong with one particular argument against abortion. For all we have seen so far, there may be other, successful, arguments against abortion. Thomson knows this perfectly well; and indeed, she says that her defence of abortion "begins" only after she has covered the ground we have considered so far.[9] Our purposes here do not require us to work through her whole defence of abortion, which is complex and very interesting. But it will be useful to look at a couple more of the imaginary stories that she employs. For they will show us the need to think carefully and critically about the argumentative work to which they are being put.

In her defence of abortion (which presumes throughout that the foetus is a person), Thomson reviews a number of different kinds of situation in which an abortion might be sought. One of those is the situation in which the pregnancy could be fatal to the mother, and in which abortion would be sought in order to save the mother's life. (Let us also presume that the foetus could be saved if the abortion is not performed.) Is abortion permissible in this situation?

Thomson points out that someone might here argue *against* abortion along the following lines. The foetus and the mother are both persons with the right to life. Each life is at stake. Each of the parties is quite innocent. A disinterested third party – the doctor – has no basis to intervene on behalf of one party against the other. He or she must remain impartial. So the doctor has no justification for performing an abortion (which would be an intervention on the mother's behalf, against the foetus).

And Thomson responds by claiming that this is a bad argument. For, she claims, it omits a very important fact. She first tells us an imaginary story in order to describe an analogous situation:

> Suppose you find yourself trapped in a tiny house with a growing child. I mean a very tiny house, and a rapidly growing child – you are already up against the wall of the house and in a few minutes you'll be crushed to death. The child on the other hand won't be crushed to death; if nothing is done to stop him from growing he'll be hurt, but in the end he'll simply burst open the house and walk out a free man.[10]

And then Thomson goes on to point out the fact so far omitted from that story: "… what we have to keep in mind is that the mother and the unborn child are not like two tenants in a small house which has, by an unfortunate mistake, been rented to both: the mother *owns* the house."[11]

The important further fact is that the mother *owns her body*. Her body is what each of the two innocently threatened parties needs in order to survive. But it is *her* body; and this gives the disinterested third party a basis on which to intervene. It is this fact, argues Thomson, which

> lets us see that a third party who says "I cannot choose between you" is fooling himself if he thinks this is impartiality. If Jones has found and fastened on a certain coat, which he needs to keep him from freezing, but which Smith also needs to keep him from freezing, then it is not impartiality that says "I cannot choose between you" when Smith owns the coat. Women have said again and again "This body is *my* body!" and they have reason to feel angry, reason to feel that it has been like shouting into the wind. Smith, after all, is hardly likely to bless us if we say to him, "Of course it's your coat, anybody would grant that it is. But no one may choose between you and Jones who is to have it."[12]

Thomson's argument, then, is that the third party is entitled to save the life of the person to whom the needed body belongs. Each of the innocent and endangered mother and foetus needs that body for survival, but the body is owned by the mother. And Thomson's two imaginary examples – the house needed by both mother and child, but owned by the mother; and the coat needed by both Smith and Jones, but owned by Smith – are provided in order to illustrate the point. Is this a good argument, and are those two imaginary illustrations playing a proper role?

Some people will feel uncomfortable with Thomson's insistence that each of us *owns* our body. They will feel that ownership is not quite the right notion to employ here. They may feel this because they believe that our body – our very bodily existence – is a *gift* from God. And that it is a gift given to us as a kind of *trust*: we are given this gift for our own flourishing and in order to love and serve others, and we are accountable to God for the way we use it. Now Thomson may have this kind of theological view in mind when she goes on to say:

> I suppose that in some views of human life the mother's body is only on loan to her, the loan not being one which gives her any prior claim to it. One who held this view might well think it impartiality to say "I cannot choose" [between mother and foetus]. But I shall simply ignore this possibility. My own view is that if a human being has any just, prior claim to anything at all, he has a just, prior claim to his own body.[13]

If Thomson is here responding to that theological view about our bodies, then her response is nothing but a bald dismissal of the view, without any argument against it and without any consideration of the philosophical role it might play. "I shall simply ignore this possibility." This will, of course, be regarded as utterly unsatisfactory by those who are inclined to hold that view; and by those who, whether or not they hold the view, would wish to explore its implications for our ethical discussion.

But we may still feel uncomfortable about the notion of ownership of our bodies without being moved by theological considerations. For though it would appear to be true that I am more closely related to my body than to anything else, it is also true that I do not come to own my body in any of the ways in which I come to own other things. My body is not something to which I *gain title*. I don't *make* it for myself. (I might feed it and look after it and help it to grow, but it is already mine long before I start to do any of those things.) I don't *buy* it, or acquire it through any kind of formal or informal exchange. I might feel that I am *given* it – though, as we have noted, Thomson appears to want to dismiss any thought of a gift which entails responsibilities to the giver. And in any case, it could not be a gift given to me in the way that other gifts are given to me, for before receiving *this* gift, I do not exist in a way that would enable me to receive anything. The gift of my body is the gift of my very existence. The possession of my body *is* my existence – my existence as an embodied individual in the world. And if we don't like the notion of gift here, then we will need to say that my body is just something that I am *naturally landed with*. I possess my body just by naturally coming into existence; my body is my natural means or place of life, of survival. Still, even though ownership seems in many ways to be a misleading notion when applied to our relation to our body, Thomson is surely right to insist on the obvious point that my body is *mine*, not yours, and vice versa. My body is *my* natural embodiment, my natural place and means of life and survival, not yours. And yours is yours, not mine.

But even if we concede to Thomson that we own our bodies in this special and very particular sense, does her argument work? She is arguing that, though both mother and foetus are persons, each with the right to life, and though each is innocent, and the life of each is at stake, the third party can perform an abortion, deciding to save the mother rather than the foetus, because the mother owns the body. The mother owns the thing each needs in order to survive. But to point this out is not yet to say enough for the argument to work. For in order to argue successfully that the third party is entitled to intervene on the mother's behalf, Thomson needs to show that there is *a relevant difference between the mother and the foetus*. And telling us that the mother owns the body does not tell us that there is a relevant *difference* unless we are *also* told that the foetus *does not* own the body. But does Thomson manage to show us *this*?

It seems to me that Thomson does not even consider this point. The question does not even arise in her discussion. She simply presumes that she has shown us a relevant difference between mother and foetus by pointing to the mother's ownership of the body. Thus she is simply taking it for granted that the mother's ownership is a sole ownership. And her imaginary examples display this presupposition. The house is owned by the mother and *not* the child. The coat is owned by Smith and *not* by Jones. But is Thomson – are we – entitled merely to take it for granted that the foetus does not *also* own the body?

Now this question may, of course, seem very odd. In what sense could it possibly be true that the foetus also – along with the mother – owns the mother's body? I stressed a moment ago that my body is mine, not yours, and vice versa. And that is surely true for the ordinary case. But pregnancy is a unique situation; and could it be unique not least because it is unlike that ordinary case? Could it be a situation in which that otherwise ordinary rule does not apply? Now we might object to this suggestion by pointing out that the mother was "in" her body long before the foetus was (and, if all goes well for her, will continue to be "in" her body long after the foetus is). It was *her* body long before it could have been the foetus's (and, all being well, will continue to be hers long after it could be the foetus's). But the question should be whether it is also the foetus's body *for the period of pregnancy*. Could it be true that the foetus, along with the mother, owns the mother's body *during that period*?

Again, we might object. For even as we confine our view to the period of pregnancy, we need to note that the mother – unlike the foetus – is responsible for the body, and can look after it in the way that the foetus cannot. But this cannot establish that the foetus does not also own the body, for we have already recognised that my body was mine long before I could take any responsibility for it. It is also true that the foetus has not *gained title* to the body in any of the ways in which we normally gain title to the things we own. But as we have seen, just the same is true of the mother and her relation to her body. She has simply been naturally landed with her body. Her embodiment is the gift of her existence – or if you prefer, her natural place or means of life, of survival. Her body is where she naturally belongs. But the very same things are true of the foetus (for the period of pregnancy): it has just been naturally landed with its connection to the mother's body; this is its embodiment, its natural place or means of life and survival. The mother's body is where the foetus naturally belongs. So, though it is certainly true to say that it is the mother's body, is it (for the period of pregnancy) any less true to say that it is also the foetus's body? The very considerations which entitle us to say that the body is *the mother's* seem also to entitle us to say that the body is *the foetus's*. And so, if we should be talking of ownership here at all, shouldn't we be talking of *joint ownership*? Shouldn't we be saying that, during the period of pregnancy, the body is owned jointly by mother and foetus? And if we should be saying this, then Thomson has not identified a relevant difference between mother and foetus, and her argument collapses.

If her argument is to work, Thomson must show us that we should dismiss the possibility of joint ownership of the body. But she does not even consider that possibility. And it seems to me that it would be very difficult to fill this gap in her argument, for, as we have seen, any ground for saying that the mother owns the body seems also to be ground for saying that the foetus similarly owns the body.

Furthermore, we can now see that Thomson's imaginary examples can here cloud our view of the logic of the question. For each of them – the house, and the coat – involves *sole ownership* of the thing that both parties need in order to survive. Her examples are not analogous to what could be the real situation, in which the parties jointly own what is needed for survival. And this is a case in which the possible disanalogies certainly do matter. For here Thomson is using her examples to illustrate how a third party would be justified in intervening on behalf of the person who owns what is needed, and her stories are therefore very misleading if the situation which they are supposed to illuminate for us – pregnancy – may lack the very feature which is critical to her argument. If we accept Thomson's stories as proper examples of the point she wants to make, in the way she intends us to accept them, then we have already taken for granted that ownership of the body can only be sole ownership; and in doing this, we have failed to recognise what Thomson really *needs* to establish, and we will fail to recognise that it looks very unlikely that she would be *able* to establish this. So we have here a case in which imaginary examples can lead us badly astray.

But I am afraid it is not the only such case, as we shall now see.

Thomson goes on to consider the kind of situation in which the pregnancy does not threaten the mother's life, and asks whether abortion would be permissible here. (We are still presuming that the foetus is a person, with the right to life.) It might well seem that in this kind of situation, the foetus's right to life does entail that an abortion would be wrong; for this right is no longer in conflict with the mother's right to life, but only with the mother's right to determine what happens in and to her body. And surely a right to life does outweigh a right to decide what happens in and to one's body. But Thomson argues that this line of reasoning is mistaken. What matters, she argues, is not merely whether the foetus has the right to life. If an abortion is to breach the foetus's rights, the foetus needs *also* to possess the particular right *to use the mother's body*. If the foetus does possess that particular right, then it is being treated unjustly if it is deprived of its place in the mother's body. But if it does not possess that particular right, then in being expelled it is not being deprived of anything to which it has any right. If we accept Thomson's argument here, the critical question now becomes: does the foetus possess that further particular right? And this is Thomson's response to that question:

> I suppose we may take it as a datum that in a case of pregnancy due to rape the mother has not given the unborn person a right to the use of her body for food and shelter. Indeed, in what pregnancy could it be supposed that the mother has given the unborn person such a right? It is not as if there were unborn persons drifting about the world, to whom a woman who wants a child says "I invite you in."[14]

What Thomson is clearly presupposing here is that if the foetus *did* have this further particular right to the use of the mother's body, it would be because the mother had *granted it* this right. And so Thomson is showing, once again, that she fails to recognise the possibility we have just been discussing – the possibility that the foetus possesses the right to be in and to use the mother's body just because this is its natural place and means of survival. Thomson is failing to recognise the possibility (which, again, she would need to argue against, if her defence of abortion is to succeed) that the foetus could possess this required further right simply naturally, as a natural right, and not because the mother has done any particular granting. (Of course, we may feel very deeply uncomfortable with the suggestion that in a pregnancy due to rape, the foetus has a *right* to be in the mother's body. But still, the general question of a natural right is one that Thomson ought to consider.) So there is once again a gap in Thomson's argument. Nevertheless, for the purposes of the discussion, let us put this gap aside and allow the presupposition she makes – that, for the foetus to possess the right to use the mother's body, it would need to be granted this right by the mother. And let us ask Thomson's question with her: in what pregnancy could it be supposed that the mother has given the unborn person such a right?

Many people will find this question less silly than Thomson appears to regard it. For, they will suggest, if we are supposed to think of the foetus as a person, then we can properly suppose that (at least in many cases) it *has* been granted the right to use the mother's body. In order for the mother to give the foetus this right, there do not need to be "unborn persons drifting about the world", to one of whom the mother says, "I invite you in." Rather, she can give the foetus this right *implicitly*, or *in effect*, by virtue of what she does given what she knows. For – presuming that she is an ordinary person with ordinary knowledge, and that she is acting voluntarily – her engagement in sexual intercourse occurs in the knowledge that pregnancy could result. If pregnancy does occur, then she is responsible for the presence within her body of a person; and doesn't that person thereby gain the right to be there? (Of course, the mother is only *partly* responsible. If her actions do give the unborn person rights against her, the actions of the other responsible party – the father – surely give the unborn person rights against him too.)

Thomson acknowledges that she needs to consider this possibility. And she concedes that it *might* turn out that there are *some* cases in which the unborn person has in this way come to possess a right to the use of the mother's body – and in which abortion would accordingly be wrong. But she does not concede that it is clear that there is *any* case in which such a right does arise in that way.[15] And to support this, she brings on another series of imaginary stories:

> For there are cases and cases, and the details make a difference. If the room is stuffy, and I therefore open a window to air it, and a burglar climbs in, it would be absurd to say, "Ah, now he can stay, she's given him a right to the use of her house – for she is partially responsible for his presence there, having voluntarily done what enabled him to get in, in full knowledge that there are such things as burglars, and that burglars burgle." It would be still more absurd to say this if I had had bars installed outside my windows, precisely to prevent burglars from getting in, and a burglar got in only because of a defect in the bars. It remains equally absurd if we imagine it is not a burglar who climbs in, but an innocent person who blunders or falls in...[16]

Thomson is performing more thought experiments. She is focusing upon the argument that through the mother's voluntary knowing activity, the foetus is given the right to use the mother's body, and putting this argument to the test by seeing whether it leads to false conclusions in imaginary cases. And she concludes that the argument fails, at least in many cases, for it leads in fact to "absurd" conclusions. Her own argument is a ***reductio ad absurdum*** of the argument she is putting to the test. (She is seeking to prove that that argument is bad by demonstrating that it leads to, or can be reduced to, absurdity.) The *reductio* has a modus tollens form, and can be expressed along the following kind of lines:

> *If the argument being considered is sound then in the imagined cases the burglar and the innocent person are granted the right to use the house. It is false (it would be absurd to claim) that the burglar and the innocent person in those cases are granted the right to use the house. Therefore, the argument being considered is not sound.*

We know that this argument form is valid. But are Thomson's premises true? Let's examine her experiments.

Should Thomson be considering *burglars* here? If we are to think of the foetus as a person, then we must consider it to be an innocent person. It has no guilty intent in occupying the mother's body; in fact, it has no intent at all. Whereas a burglar is *purposely intruding* on the property, with *guilty intent*. The burglar *knows* that he has no right to be on the property. Now Thomson might respond by insisting that this disanalogy with pregnancy does not matter. For, she can say, she is putting a *particular principle* to the test – namely, the principle that I have given someone the right to use my property if I am (to use her words) partially responsible for his presence there, having voluntarily done what enabled him to get in, in full knowledge that someone could get in in that way. That principle, Thomson might add, is what is being relied upon by the person who argues that the foetus is granted by the mother the right to the use of her body; and the thought experiment shows that the principle is false. Now I think that Thomson is right to claim that she has shown that *that principle* is incorrect. With the case of the burglar, she has provided what we call a ***counter-example*** to the principle. The principle states that something will be true when certain conditions are fulfilled. And Thomson has displayed a case in which those conditions *have* been fulfilled (I have voluntarily done what has enabled someone to be on my property, knowing that this could happen), but in which what is said will then be true is in fact *false* (that person has *not* gained the right to be there). And so the principle – as a general moral principle – is incorrect, for it does not hold true in all cases as a general principle needs to do. So far, so good. But is *that* principle the principle which Thomson ought to be testing?

It is not, in fact, the relevant principle. The person who argues that the mother in effect grants the foetus the right to use her body will, of course, be relying on the fact that the foetus – unlike the burglar – is innocent. Now Thomson does go on, as we have seen, to introduce this consideration into her thought experiment. She does so in the briefest terms, asserting that it is just as absurd to claim that the right to use the house has been given to "an innocent person who blunders or falls in" as it is to claim that the burglar has been given that right. But this description of the innocent person does not yet provide a proper analogy with pregnancy. The foetus does not "blunder in" to the mother's body; it has not made any mistake. And as Hursthouse points out in her discussion of Thomson's argument, a further vital consideration has so far been omitted. The foetus is analogous not to any ordinary innocent person, but to an innocent person *who needs to stay in the house in order to survive*.[17] The ordinary innocent person who blunders into my house can recognise his mistake and recognise that he does not belong there; he can be politely shown the door, and all will be well. But the foetus is in the mother's body not because of any mistake of its own, and to remove it from there would be *to kill it*. The person arguing that the foetus has gained the right to stay will wish to rely upon this as an essential point. It is a point which can be built into the *relevant* moral principle, which might now go something like this:

> *If I voluntarily did something which could enable someone to come perfectly innocently and naturally onto my property, and as a result of what I did a person* did *come onto my property perfectly innocently and naturally, and this person would be* killed *if I now removed him from my property, and I knew that all of this could be the outcome of what I did when I voluntarily did it, then I bear responsibility for that person's being on my property, and he has gained the right to stay in order to survive*.

(And the principle could add that my partner in our voluntary activity also shares responsibility for that person.) *That* principle appears, I think, to be a much more plausible principle. It seems to me that it would be very far from "absurd" to claim that under such conditions, the innocent person has gained the right to remain. And *if* we are to regard the foetus as a person, and if we are to regard the mother's body as like a house which she owns, then it is a principle which applies to pregnancy, and which appears to show that in many cases the mother does indeed in effect grant to the foetus the right to use her body, and that in those cases abortion would therefore be wrong.

And Thomson's thought experiments are quite irrelevant to *that* principle. Her imaginary stories do *not* provide counter-examples to that principle, for they do not fulfil the conditions specified by the principle. (They do not describe situations in which an innocent person quite blamelessly arrives on the property and needs to stay there in order to survive.) So the thought experiments do *not* show what Thomson intends them to show – that there are some cases in which the foetus does not come to gain the right to use the mother's body in the argued-for way. Indeed, here, as previously, Thomson's illustrations are positively misleading. For they are disanalogous to pregnancy, and the disanalogies are crucially important. (The person who argues that the foetus is in effect granted the right to use the mother's body can insist that it is essential to the argument that the foetus is an innocent person, arriving in the body by perfectly natural means, and that his expulsion from the body would be the cause of his death.) If we accept Thomson's stories as legitimate illustrations of the situation we need to consider, we will fail to see crucial points upon which the argument she is attacking depends.

Thomson's thought experiments, then, are in fact a mixed bag. Some are genuinely useful. Others fail to do the work she intends and can actually lead us astray. But either way, we can learn from them. In the one kind of case, we see how imagination can be employed to produce a telling counter-example to an argument or principle – demonstrating that the argument is bad, or that the principle is incorrect. In the other kind of case, we see the need to exercise great care in critically examining any alleged counter-example. Is it a *genuine* counter-example? Does it lack features which are crucial to the real issue? Does it import features which don't belong? And so on.

Because it contains those and other flaws, I believe that Thomson's defence of abortion fails.[18] If this verdict is correct, must we say that abortion is wrong after all? Once again, the answer is No. We have been finding faults in Thomson's *arguments*. But bad arguments might have true conclusions. (Indeed, would we wish to oppose Thomson's conclusions that abortion would be justified when otherwise the pregnancy would kill the mother, or in the case of "a sick and desperately frightened fourteen-year-old schoolgirl, pregnant due to rape"?)[19] Once again, however, the arguer needs to go back to the drawing board. But we may well also find that our criticisms of Thomson's arguments have produced plenty of material upon which we can reflect in thinking about the morality of abortion, and which can help us to work towards positive conclusions.

Conclusion

There is a great deal more to the study of logic than we have covered in this chapter. But we have gathered some important tools and watched them at work. We have seen how to *identify* an argument, by putting it in *standard form*. We have seen that, in order to *evaluate* an argument, we need to ask *whether it is valid* and *whether its premises are true*. We have noted the particular roles of arguments that have *conditional* premises. We have seen where the *consequences* of some view might, and where they might not, *put that view to the test*. We have seen how *imagination* can be used to construct *thought experiments* which allow us to test arguments or principles; but we have also witnessed the need to examine those thought experiments very *critically* – taking great care to ensure that we are not misled by them.

We will employ these tools at various places in the following chapters of this book. But more importantly, they are tools we will find useful as we think carefully and critically about the moral views we need to consider – our own views and those of others – throughout our professional lives.

Notes

1 Rosalind Hursthouse, *Beginning Lives* (Blackwell/Open University, Oxford, 1987). Hursthouse discusses this argument on pages 32 to 38.
2 Peter Singer advances similar arguments in his *Practical Ethics* (Cambridge University Press, Cambridge, 1979), pp. 108–10.
3 Hursthouse discusses this view in *Beginning Lives* (Hursthouse, *op. cit.*, pp. 47–59).
4 The likelihoods I have crudely described can be formulated as the elements required for the application of Bayes's Theorem.
5 Judith Jarvis Thomson, "A Defense of Abortion", in *Philosophy and Public Affairs*, Vol. 1, No. 1, pp. 47–66.
6 *Ibid.*, p. 48.
7 *Ibid.*, pp. 48–9.
8 Hursthouse offers a very interesting discussion of this case, and considers what our actual duties towards the violinist might be. She agrees with Thomson that the violinist has no *right* to stay hooked up to you, but she is more inclined than is Thomson to recognise that you also have other moral duties in this situation – duties which flow from a variety of virtues, not merely the virtue of justice (which is concerned with rights). She considers how those duties might alter depending upon *how much* you need to do in order to save the violinist's life. And she concludes: "I am not sure what I think about the violinist case, but I am sure that the more I make it akin to the average pregnancy (I am not bed-ridden, can lead my normal life for a lot of the nine months, etc.) the more certain I become that anyone who finds themselves in the violinist situation *is* morally required to put up with it; that it would be callous, or cowardly, or self-indulgent or self-centred to refuse cold-bloodedly." (*Op. cit.*, p. 203)
9 *Ibid.*, p. 50.
10 *Ibid.*, p. 52.
11 *Ibid.*, p. 53.
12 *Ibid.*, pp. 53–4.
13 *Ibid.*, p. 54.
14 *Ibid.*, p. 57.
15 "It seems to me that the argument we are looking at can establish at most that there are *some* cases in which the unborn person has a right to the use of its mother's body,

and therefore *some* cases in which abortion is unjust killing. There is room for much discussion and argument as to precisely which, if any." *Ibid.*, p. 59.

16 *Ibid.*, pp. 58–9.

17 Hursthouse, *op. cit.*, pp. 188–9. Hursthouse offers her own illuminating thought experiment which does address this essential consideration. And she criticises another of Thomson's thought experiments – concerning "people-seeds".

18 As I have mentioned, Thomson seeks to defend abortion for a series of different kinds of situation. Her defences, and my reasons for rejecting them, can be very briefly summarised as follows. First, she considers the situation in which the pregnancy threatens the mother's life, and asks whether the mother *herself* would be entitled to perform an abortion in order to save her own life. Her answer seems to be that it is simply *obvious* that the mother is entitled to do this. And she mentions in this connection *self-defence*. But many people will here feel that, if we are indeed required to think of the foetus as *a person*, it is not *simply obvious* that the mother is entitled to perform an abortion. They will feel, rather, that the situation presents an agonising moral dilemma. And reference to self-defence is out of place here, for the moral doctrine of self-defence applies in situations where the person threatening one's life is doing so *intentionally* (or at least recklessly), and of course the foetus has no such intention. Secondly, Thomson argues that a third party (a doctor) would be entitled to perform an abortion to save the mother's life, because the mother owns the body. But as we have discussed, Thomson fails to show that the foetus does not also own the body. Thirdly, Thomson argues that, in situations in which the mother's life is not at stake, abortion is not a breach of the foetus's *rights* because, at least in many cases, it has no right to the use of the mother's body. But as we have discussed, she fails to show that, at least in many cases, the foetus has not in effect been granted that right by the mother's voluntary activity. And fourthly, Thomson argues that an abortion would not be a breach of the mother's *duties of charity* – or, as Thomson prefers to call them, duties of decency – for those duties do not require the mother to make the kinds of sacrifice which would be entailed by going through a pregnancy. But there are good reasons to respond that our duties of charity can under certain circumstances be considerably more rigorous than Thomson recognises. Hursthouse lists a number of situations where it seems clear that we could be required by charity to make large sacrifices in order to sustain a person's life. (Hursthouse, *op. cit.*, pp. 198–204.)

19 Thomson, *op. cit.*, p. 65.

3
Is morality relative?

At the end of Chapter One, we heard the objection that morality is merely subjective or relative – an objection which, if correct, would suggest that the study of ethics is rather pointless. We are now ready to return to that objection and consider whether it is indeed correct. But before we go any further, let's note that, in our discussion throughout Chapter Two, we have been presuming that there is truth to be sought in ethics – truth which each of us ought to recognise as truth. We have been asking whether particular moral arguments have true conclusions, whether a certain moral view can be shown to be false, and so on. These have seemed to be perfectly proper questions; and by pursuing them, we have already achieved fruitful results. Among other things, we have surely recognised some arguments as having true conclusions, and that some views are to be rejected as unacceptable – as views which each of us ought to recognise as false. So our working assumption that there is objective truth to be sought in ethics has already proved to be very illuminating. It would take a lot, I think, to convince us that all of this has been thoroughly misguided. However, with that noted, let us now turn to consider directly the claim that we are mistaken to suppose that there is objective truth in ethics.

The objection left hanging at the end of Chapter One ran together a number of different claims. The objector drew our attention to the controversial nature of morality, and to the differences in moral views. It was pointed out that we find different moral beliefs and feelings and attitudes across different groups and cultures. In particular, it was claimed that the moral views of so-called religious people differ from those of so-called non-religious people. And the conclusion was drawn that morality is relative, or subjective, and therefore that it is mistaken to think that ethics can seek to study objective moral truths, for there are no such things.

We need to sort out what is going on in that line of thinking.

DOI: 10.4324/9781003176541-4

What does it mean to say that morality is relative?

Let's start with the radical conclusion – namely, that morality is relative, or subjective. Those terms ("relative" and "subjective") tend be used more or less interchangeably within popular discussion of these matters. There are proper philosophical reasons for distinguishing these terms; but for our purposes here, we need not worry too much about the precise and different senses in which the terms should be used. The important point is that they are both being used in contrast to the term "objective", and *that* term is being used to describe a certain kind of truth. What kind of truth? Let's consider some examples. In the front garden of the house opposite mine, there is (I assure you) a particular area within which there are eight separate rocks, each of a mass greater than ten kilograms. It is *true* that those rocks are there, and this is an *objective* truth. It is not a truth which is dependent upon me in any way; nor is it dependent upon how anyone is feeling, or on what anyone is experiencing or believing. It is a fact *out there*, as it were – a fact about the independent, objective world. And it happens to be a truth that I can *know*. (I am looking at those rocks now, through the window of my study.) And similarly, anyone else, properly situated in relation to those rocks, could know this truth. (There are very important philosophical questions about how we can really know facts about the world external to our own minds, but those are questions for a different book.) But not all objective truths are known. On the surface of the moon right now, there is a certain number of separate rocks each of a mass greater than ten kilograms. I don't know what that number is, and I suppose that no other human being knows that number. Perhaps no-one will ever know. But, whatever that number is, it is an objective truth that there is that number of rocks there now. People might believe, or have some feeling which causes them to believe, that the number is such and such; but this would not *make it the case* that the number is what they believe. Nor does it *cease* to be true that the number is what it is just because no-one believes it or has any feelings about it at all. It is a truth about what is out there, on the surface of the moon; it is not a truth about *us*. We may not come to know what that number is, but we can certainly be *mistaken* about it, for we could believe the wrong thing. (Perhaps I dream a number; or perhaps some scientist announces the conclusion of a miscalculation, and I come to believe what is announced.) The fact about that number is a fact which is independent of what anyone believes or feels.

In the same way, when it is said that morality is objective, it is being claimed that moral truths are independent of what anyone believes or feels. And they are truths that we might get right or wrong; we may be correct or incorrect in our moral beliefs. We don't usually talk of objective truths as being true *for* someone or other; but if we were to use that kind of language, we would need to say that objective truths are true *for us all.* They are universal truths, or truths for everyone, whether we know them or not, and whether we like it or not. (There are important philosophical questions about whether it is correct to think of morality in terms of *truths*. For instance, much morality seems to consist of *rules* – for example, "Don't steal" or "Love your neighbour as yourself" – and we don't say that a rule is *true*, or false. I could perfectly sensibly say that the remark "There are eight rocks over there" is true. But I could not sensibly say that the remark "Don't steal" is true. However, we might say that a rule such as "Don't steal" is *correct* – that it is correctly expressing an obligation, or that it is properly binding, or something like that. And we might say that whether it is correct or not is an *objective* matter. And in any case, we do make many moral judgements as if we are making claims about what is *true*. For instance, we say that we ought not to steal, and that murder is wrong, and that we ought to love our neighbours as ourselves, and so on. And these certainly seem to be claims that we can regard as objectively true, or false. We can certainly believe that it is true that we ought not to steal, and that it is true that murder is wrong, and that we ought to love our neighbours as ourselves.)

But then, what does it mean to claim that morality is subjective or relative? Think again about the rocks. If we ask how many rocks of that mass there are in that space across the road, or on the surface of the moon, we are asking a question to which there is an objectively true answer. We may or may not be able to know that answer; we might be mistaken about it. But there is a right answer – an answer which is right regardless of what any of us believes or fails to believe. However, contrast some other questions. Suppose I ask on what side of the road I ought to drive. The answer I receive will depend upon the country I am in. In some countries, I will be told to drive on the left side of the road; in others, on the right. Or suppose I ask what is the most delicious dessert. The answer will depend upon those whom I ask. Some people will say that it is one thing (chocolate ice cream, strawberries and cream, etc.); some will say something else (pavlova topped with cream and banana and passionfruit, apple pie and custard, etc.). But now suppose that, hearing all those different answers, I insist on asking what is *really* the correct side of the road to drive on, or what is *truly* the most delicious dessert. It will be pointed out that I am confused. Even though they are different, each of the answers I have heard can be correct, and I am confused about the kind of truth that makes them correct or incorrect. The right answer concerning the side of the road depends on the particular convention in the nation for which I am asking the question. A country can decide that people there are to drive on the right, or on the left, and this decision, or convention, will then give rise to the relevant law in that country. But countries can decide this question either way, so the answer to my question will depend upon the particular country. The correctness of that answer will be *relative to* the particular country. (The answer "Drive on the left" will be correct relative to Australia, but incorrect relative to Italy. It will be right *for* Australia, but wrong *for* Italy.) And if I insist on asking "But what's the right answer *full stop?*", "What's the right answer *for everyone?*", it will be pointed out that I am confused in imagining that the truth in question is an objective or universal or absolute truth, whereas in fact it is a relative truth. (There is an objectively correct answer to the question concerning the correct side on which to drive *in Italy*, but it is correct because of a truth merely *about Italy*. It is a truth for Italy to *decide*. And other countries can decide the question for themselves in different ways.) Similarly, the answers concerning the most delicious dessert depend upon the particular tastes and preferences of the people whom I ask. Tastes are *subjective* – they depend upon the particular subject, the person, whose taste we are asking about.[1] And because tastes vary, different people can be correctly reporting their own preferences even though their reports differ from the reports of others. ("Pavlova" is the true answer for Agatha; "strawberries" is the true answer for Bertram.) So again, the truth about the most delicious dessert is a subjective truth, relative to each particular person. And if I insist on asking about the most delicious dessert *for everyone*, then I am confused about the kind of truth in question.

So when it is said that morality is relative or subjective, it is being claimed that moral requirements depend upon particular persons, or cultures. Whether something is morally right or wrong will depend upon the particular person or culture for whom that question is asked. What is right *for this* person or culture may be wrong *for that* person or culture. And there is no such thing as what is morally binding *for all* cultures, or all people. To think that there is such a thing would be confused: it would be to imagine that moral requirements are stated by objective (or universal) truths, whereas they are merely relative.

That, then, is what it *means* to claim that morality is relative. But now, is that claim *correct?*

The bad argument for believing that morality is relative

What reason can be given for claiming that morality is relative? The reasoning we have heard in support of this claim simply appeals to the divergences between the moral views of different people and different cultures across history and across the world, so we can summarise it by a very simple argument:

> *Different people and different cultures have different moral views.*
>
> ---
>
> *Morality is relative (to particular people and cultures).*

That is indeed a simple argument, containing only a single premise. So we can straightforwardly apply to it those tools of critical reasoning we gathered in the previous chapter. We need to ask whether the argument is sound, and we do this by asking whether it is valid, and whether its premise is true.

So, is the argument valid? I am afraid that the argument falls at this first hurdle, for the fact (if it is a fact) that different people have different views on some matter does not show that there is no such thing as objective truth on that matter, as we can immediately recognise when we consider any of countless examples.

For instance, over the course of my lecturing career, I have had occasion to set very many examinations. Each exam question is designed to test whether the student has learned some particular material required for the course. I am sorry to report that I sometimes receive a wide divergence of answers to a particular question. Nevertheless, this does not convince me that I am simply confused in marking some of those answers as wrong (and many, I am relieved to note, as correct). And suppose a student comes to see me to appeal against his failing grade. I will listen carefully to his protest. But let's suppose that his complaint goes along the following lines. He points out that different students offered different answers to the exam questions, and he argues that this shows that there were no objectively correct answers and so his answers should not be marked as wrong because relative to him they were right. I am afraid that this argument will not advance his cause one bit. His exam result will not be altered and he will be told to go back and learn the course material – and to start working on his skills in critical reasoning.

Or think yet again of the question of the number of rocks greater than ten kilograms on the moon. Let's suppose that scientists turn their minds to that question. They might develop theories which allow them to make predictions concerning that number of rocks. And – as often happens in science – their predictions turn out to vary, perhaps very widely. But nobody would conclude that therefore there is no such thing as the objective truth concerning the number of rocks of that mass on the surface of the moon.

What is reported in the premise of the argument – the differences between moral views – is consistent with a number of possibilities. It is consistent with the possibility that morality is indeed relative – that moral views are true only relatively to the particular people or cultures holding those views. But it is *also* consistent with the possibility that there is objective truth in morality, but that many views diverge from that truth. It is consistent with the possibility that some of us are mistaken in our moral beliefs. The truth of the premise would not show us that one rather than the other of those possibilities is true. So it is *not* the case that *if it were true* that different people and cultures hold different moral views *then it would have to be true* that morality is relative. The argument is invalid.

So that argument for moral relativism – the view that holds that morality is relative – is unsound. But before we leave the argument, it is interesting to consider whether it fulfils the other requirement for soundness. Is the premise of the argument *true?*

The premise is, of course, true as a description of the range of moral views we actually observe. But what do we see if we drill down to the more basic principles and attitudes underlying those various views? Let's consider a case of the general kind that has led numerous social scientists to conclude that morality is relative to particular cultures. Suppose that anthropologists discover a tribe in Africa that displays what seems to us to be very extraordinary behaviour. When the boys within this tribe approach their adolescent years, they are mutilated in various ways by the elders in their tribe (the scars of these wounds will remain on their bodies as long as they live), and then they are driven out of the tribal communities and left to fend for themselves in the wilderness. If they manage to survive for a lengthy period, they will then be readmitted into the tribal community from which they were banished. Some of the boys die: they bleed to death, or their wounds become infected, or they perish through thirst or hunger or exposure. And those who manage to survive do so only at the cost of considerable pain and suffering. The anthropologists observe these practices and remark on how greatly this tribal morality differs from our morality. *We* believe that we owe duties of care to the members of our community – not least to the younger members of our community. We believe that we ought not to harm them, and we certainly ought not to kill them, or allow them to die. We believe that we should provide social arrangements within which our younger members can grow into the healthy maturity in which they can flourish. But this tribe (the anthropologists report) clearly does not share those attitudes. It engages in practices which lead to the death of some of their boys and which cause very painful bodily harm and suffering to all of them. Wounded as they are, the boys are then abandoned by the community. And whether they are eventually allowed to return to the community depends on whether they manage to survive without any community care at all.

But now let's suppose that some rather more thoughtful members of the anthropological team take the time and make the effort to learn the language of that tribe and to earn its trust, and thereby equip themselves to enquire about the tribal practices. And thus they learn that those practices constitute traditional rites of passage for the male members of the tribe. They learn that this tradition is cherished because it is firmly believed to promote what both the boys and the wider tribal community need. For the tribe believes that, in the harsh conditions under which it lives in the African bush, its male members will lack the fortitude and endurance and skill to survive and to support the whole community unless they learn to overcome these trials of pain and suffering and physical hardship. Tribal elders explain that the whole tribe grieves if a boy dies; but that the trials are necessary to help the boys grow into full vigorous maturity – the maturity in which they can flourish as individuals, and take their rightful part in leading and protecting the whole community. The elders explain that in treating the boys in this way, they are seeking to discharge their sacred duty to provide true, effective care for the younger members of the community (and so in turn for the wider community).

What have the anthropologists now discovered? They have learned, of course, that the tribe seeks to justify its practices by appeal to deep moral principles which are just like those to which we appeal. The tribal elders appeal to their duty of care towards the young members of the community. They believe that, though they are doing bodily harm to their boys, they are nevertheless acting for the boys' overall good. They believe that their practices provide the means through which their boys can truly attain their proper maturity and thus be equipped to live a flourishing life. The anthropologists have in fact discovered that the tribe's moral views and our moral views are *not* different – at least at this fairly fundamental level. The tribe *applies* those views in a way which is very different from the way in which we apply them. We may well believe that the tribe's practical application of those views is incorrect – in fact, dangerously incorrect. (And the tribal elders might take a critical view of the ways in which we raise our boys.) Were we to sit down with members of the tribe and address that question, there would be much room for discussion. But discussion would indeed be possible precisely because we would be operating from shared moral principles, and thus we would be in a position to reason together concerning what those principles practically entail.

And that case is similar in kind to many others which seem to indicate real moral difference. At the surface level – the level of our practical application of our moral principles – there is indeed significant difference between the moral beliefs of different people and cultures. But when we seek to expose the deeper moral principles underlying our practices, we tend to uncover principles which we share.

And we also find a recognition of generally held moral principles in places where we might least expect to find it. In the world about us, there is plenty of behaviour that we readily classify as immoral. We can observe it close at hand, in the attitudes and actions of those in our immediate sphere. Even closer to hand, dare I say it, we can observe it in our own attitudes and actions – in those attitudes and actions of which we are ashamed. (Or at least we know, if we are honest with ourselves, that they are attitudes and actions of which we *ought* to be ashamed.) But of course, we observe immorality more easily, and more comfortably for ourselves, in the more spectacular acts of wickedness elsewhere in the world. Now it is interesting to note that where we do observe it, we also hear *excuses* being offered for it. The people engaging in the immorality may be merely *pretending* that they have genuine excuses for the actions they perform, but they nevertheless make the excuses. And the important point here is that these excuses appeal to principles that we all recognise. In attempting to justify our own behaviour, we may appeal to our rights, or the demands of fairness, or our own important needs, or the claim that we were under some kind of compulsion, and so on. And we hear appeals of very similar kinds when we turn our attention to the more spectacular acts of wickedness. So for instance, an aggressive military regime invades a neighbouring country claiming that the territory really belongs to its own nation, or that it is liberating unjustly displaced people and restoring their rights by uniting them with their folk within their proper homeland. The dictator leads his forces in genocide by claiming that the community to be wiped out consists of rats and cockroaches, and that these vermin are infecting the wider society by their corruption, and thus threatening the security and health and indeed the very life of the nation. And so on. Now typically, of course, these claims are outrageously false. They are lies put up as a smokescreen for what is in fact simply wanton greed and hatred and murder and theft and power-hungry oppression. And even when those who are perpetrating these evils do to some extent believe their excuses, they may be morally blameworthy for allowing themselves to believe them – for wilfully engaging in the malicious rationalisations and self-deceptions which give rise to their beliefs. But the point is that the excuses are offered. The tyrant does not simply say, "I possess the power, I choose to use it in this way, and that's the end of the discussion." He appeals instead to moral principles that we all recognise. For we agree with him that countries possess a right to self-determination, and proper jurisdiction over their own territory. We agree that people who have been unjustly displaced should be able to return to their homeland. We agree that a nation is entitled to defend itself against a threat to its existence. We agree that rats and cockroaches and other disease-carrying animals do not possess the rights that full human beings possess. And so on. We *disagree* that those principles *apply* to the situations to which the tyrant applies them. But we accept the principles to which he appeals. And he shows, by his excuses, that he recognises those principles. So, interestingly enough, we find a common recognition of similar moral principles even in places where we find grossly objectionable activity going on – activity which we condemn as immoral.

So there appears to be good reason to hold that the premise of the argument for moral relativism is false – at least if it is taken to refer to the more fundamental moral views and principles of people and cultures. (It is important to keep in mind that we are here discussing moral *views and beliefs*, not *behaviour*. As we have just noted, there is plenty of different behaviour to be observed, including behaviour that we condemn. But the premise of the argument for moral relativism concerns what people believe, not what people do.) It is interesting to note that different people and cultures in fact share common moral views and beliefs, at least at a fairly fundamental level, and at least to some considerable extent.

But then, what should we conclude about moral relativism? We need to be careful here. What we have seen so far is that the argument we have heard for moral relativism is unsound. It is invalid, and there is reason to doubt its premise. But to show this about an argument is not yet to show anything about whether the conclusion of the argument is true or false. As we noted in Chapter Two, a bad argument could have a true conclusion. So we need to do more if we are going to be able to draw our own clear conclusion about whether moral relativism is correct or incorrect.

And here we face a real difficulty. For the question we are trying to decide here is whether there are any objective moral truths – moral truths that are true for us all. Now the most direct way to decide that question would be by producing some moral truths that we can all recognise to be objective moral truths. But this may be more difficult than it sounds. Think for a moment not about morality, but about our knowledge of the observable natural world. I gave as an example of a clear objective truth the fact that there are eight rocks of a mass greater than ten kilograms in that particular space across the road. But even a truth like that could be challenged by someone who is brazen enough to do so. "How do you *know* that?" he might insist. (And perhaps he is not merely wilfully challenging what the rest of us can see; perhaps he has some particular reason – medical or psychological or philosophical – to doubt the evidence of his eyes and other senses.) Now the fact that someone can challenge this truth does not mean that it is *not* an objective truth. But it does indicate the difficulty in pointing to truths which we can all *recognise* to be objective truths – even truths about the natural world. And the difficulty would seem to be all the greater when we are seeking moral truths. For they would not be the sort of truths that we could observe by looking at the world. Moral truths are not truths that we can *read off* the world; they are truths *against which* the world (which includes us) is *evaluated*. Moral principles are not seen *in* the world; they are the *standards by which* what *is* seen in the world is *judged* to be good or bad, right or wrong. So where, or how, can we recognise them? And how can we tell that they have objective force, and apply to us all?

The answer to that question is that there *is* something that we can see. We can see that we are *unavoidably committed* to the existence of real moral truths. For we can see that in our moral thought and talk and behaviour, we *take it for granted* that moral truths *are* objective and that there are moral standards and principles that *do* apply to us all. And this is visible in a number of different ways.

Reasons to believe that morality is not relative

First, we believe that there can be moral progress and regress. We believe that the moral views held by a person or within a society can get better or worse. We often cite the abolition of slavery as an instance of moral progress within the western nations. We believe that, in coming to accept that they ought to abolish slavery, people in Britain and elsewhere changed their attitudes for the better. And as an example of moral regress, we can cite the widespread acceptance of Hitler's policies within Germany during the 1930s. But now, what does it *mean* to say that there is moral progress or regress? Well, what does it mean when we say that I am making progress in *any* way? It means that I am getting closer to a goal, or target, or some point to which I ought to be heading. I undergo some sort of progress, or regress, when I am drawing closer to, or further away from, some significant point. But this can happen only if the point is independent of me. I can walk towards, or away from, the lamp post at the end of my street. But I can't walk towards, or away from, myself. I can make my slow progress in learning French only if there is such a thing as real fluency in French – something to which I am getting somewhat closer. Fluency in French is my target, or goal; though it is not something which I possess now. It represents a standard which is independent of me – an objective standard. And similarly, in claiming that there is moral progress or regress, we are claiming that there is movement between actual moral attitudes (the attitude towards slavery, etc.) and the independent standards against which the actual attitudes should be judged. In claiming that there is progress, we are claiming that the attitudes are drawing closer to the right standards. And in claiming that there is regress, we are claiming that they are drawing away from those standards. We are taking it for granted, in other words, that there are real, objective moral standards against which the attitudes can be assessed – real, objective standards towards which or away from which the attitudes might travel.

But this means that we are taking it for granted that moral relativism is false. For if moral relativism is correct, then there *are no* objective standards against which a person's or a culture's moral attitudes are to be assessed. The only moral standards, according to relativism, are the moral attitudes which happen to be the *actual* attitudes of that person or culture. But then there can be no question of an independent yardstick against which those attitudes can be measured. The attitudes of a society might *change*, but there can be no question of their getting closer to or further away from the standard by which they are to be assessed, for *they are* their own standard. There can be no question of their getting better or worse. "Better" and "worse" presuppose an objective standard. If relativism is correct, then to say that there is moral progress is as absurd as to say that I am walking towards myself.

But talk of moral progress, or regress, is not absurd. We firmly believe that the abolition of slavery was movement in the *right* direction, and that the acceptance of Hitler's policies was movement in the *wrong* direction. And there are countless other examples. We are committed to the objectivity of moral standards.

Now the relativist might object to this. He might say that when I judge that the abolition of slavery was an improvement, I *am* in fact assessing this societal change against a standard which is independent of that society. Nevertheless, I am doing so in a way which is consistent with relativism. For I am assessing this change against *my own* attitudes. In saying that it was an instance of moral progress, I am saying that it was a case in which the attitudes changed to become *more like my attitudes*. So I am able to evaluate the change ("Was it progress or regress?"), but I do so in a way which is still consistent with moral relativism, for I am here regarding all moral attitudes as to be assessed by comparing them to my own attitudes. I am taking it for granted, in other words, that moral attitudes are true or false *relative to me*. For after all – he might add – if *I'm* going to evaluate any attitude, I need to do so by comparing it to a standard that *I hold*, so it's got to be *my* standard.

But that is a bad objection. It is confused. From the fact that I hold to a standard, it does not follow that the standard is *merely* a standard *for me*. It may be an objective standard. (When I assess a piece of arithmetic as correct or incorrect, I am not applying my own merely relative standard.) And we can see very directly that the objection is bad by noting that I can perfectly sensibly ask whether *my own* moral attitudes might undergo change for the better or worse. I can perfectly sensibly wonder whether I myself might undergo moral progress or regress. (Of course, we are more inclined to feel that we have undergone moral progress than regress, but – as we realise when we seriously consider the possibilities – we could be fooling ourselves.) We can perfectly sensibly wonder whether our change of attitude on the issue of, say, abortion, or euthanasia, or sexual diversity really was a change in the direction of moral truth. We can perfectly sensibly ask whether we *ought* to change our attitudes on one or other of such issues. But, as we have already seen, none of those questions or wonderings can make any sense if there is no objective standard, independent of my own attitudes, against which my own attitudes are to be properly assessed. Wondering whether my own moral attitudes can change for the better or worse presupposes that there are objective moral standards. So – again – we take it for granted that relativism is not correct.

Another thing that shows us that we believe in the objectivity of morality is the fact that we have moral disagreements. Now of course, the relativist *stresses* our moral differences, so how can disagreement be an indicator of objectivity? Difference, however, is one thing; disagreement is a much more particular thing. To disagree with someone, there needs to be something we are disagreeing *about*. And the logical structure of our moral disagreements shows this. Consider the following conversation between Person A and Person B:

> A: "An abortion late in the pregnancy when neither the mother's life nor her health is at stake would be morally wrong."
>
> B: "No, that's not true! An abortion is morally permissible under any circumstances, so long as it's the mother's choice."

That conversation represents a genuine disagreement. Its logical structure is just like that of countless other disagreements we have. Imagine, for instance, two scientists, C and D, who develop theories which give different predictions of the number of rocks on the surface of the moon. Each is quite sure of her theory, and so they have a conversation in which they express their disagreement in the same sort of way as we have just seen:

> C: "The number of separate rocks with a mass greater than ten kilograms on the surface of the moon is about 100 million."
>
> D: "No, that's not true! That number is about 10 billion."

C and D are disagreeing *about the number of rocks on the moon*. A and B are disagreeing *about the circumstances in which abortion would be morally permissible*. In each case they are saying what they believe *about* something that a belief could be correct or incorrect about.

But now consider this conversation, between E and F:

> E: "The most delicious dessert is pavlova topped with cream and berries."
>
> F: "No, that's not true! The most delicious dessert is strawberries with vanilla ice cream."

If F's reply is serious, and not merely a joke, we can immediately see that it is badly confused. Her words "No, that's not true!" are out of place. In identifying the most delicious dessert, E and F are expressing their own tastes – tastes which differ. Each one's remark is really a remark *about herself* – her own taste. And when we spell that out, we can see how absurd F's reply is:

> E: "My favourite dessert is pavlova topped with cream and berries."
>
> F: "No, that's not true! My favourite dessert is strawberries with vanilla ice cream."

The words "No, that's not true!" are completely out of place because, in reporting her different preference, F is not *denying* what E is saying. Each can be correctly reporting her own preference, and those preferences differ, because E's and F's tastes differ. The conversation should go simply like this:

> E: "My favourite dessert is pavlova topped with cream and berries."
>
> F: "My favourite dessert is strawberries with vanilla ice cream."

And there we see that there is no *disagreement*, for E and F are not talking about the same thing. Each is talking about herself and her relation to a particular dessert. They are reporting and comparing their differences, but they are not disagreeing. And each report is correct, for it is true *relative to* its reporter.

But let's now imagine that moral relativism is correct. Let's imagine that a moral view is true merely relative to the person who holds that view: your views are true for you, mine are true for me. And now let's recall the original conversation between A and B, expressing a moral disagreement:

> A: "An abortion late in the pregnancy when neither the mother's life nor her health is at stake would be morally wrong."
>
> B: "No, that's not true! An abortion is morally permissible under any circumstances so long as it's the mother's choice."

If relativism is true, then A and B are each merely expressing their own attitudes – attitudes that are true merely for themselves. But in that case, their conversation has the same logical structure as the first conversation between E and F:

> E: "My favourite dessert is pavlova topped with cream and berries."
>
> F: "No, that's not true! My favourite dessert is strawberries with vanilla ice cream."

And that conversation, as we saw, is absurd. For F cannot be denying what E is asserting. They are not talking about something independent of their own individual tastes. And similarly, if moral relativism is correct, B's response to A is completely absurd. B's words "No, that's not true!" are completely misplaced. For in stating their moral views on abortion, A and B are simply reporting their own subjective attitudes to abortion. So B cannot be talking about what A is talking about. And B cannot be denying what A is asserting. And so they cannot be disagreeing with one another. If they think that they are disagreeing, then they are thoroughly confused.

But they are not confused. They really are disagreeing. And that means that they cannot be taking it for granted that their attitudes are merely true for themselves. The logical structure of their conversation cannot be like the structure of the conversation between E and F. A and B must be taking it for granted that there is something that their moral attitudes can be getting right or wrong – an objective truth against which their own attitudes are to be assessed. They are both talking *about* that objective truth, and they are disagreeing about what it is.

What's more, our moral disagreements can become vehement, even violent. Some disagreements are mild enough, or intractable enough, for us to feel that we should just tolerate them. Nevertheless, we are not prepared to tolerate every kind of different moral attitude – at least when the attitudes are expressed in actual behaviour. But this would be ridiculous if moral relativism were correct. It would be quite absurd to come to blows over the question whether pavlova or apple pie is the most delicious dessert. It would be completely idiotic to threaten another country with war because it arranges that its citizens should drive on the right side of the road, when we drive on the left. But if other attempted remedies fail, it may not be at all idiotic to threaten war against a nation carrying out a programme of genocide, or unjustly invading neighbouring countries and subjecting them to murderous tyrannical rule.

And that leads to a wider, simpler observation which shows how deeply we assume that moral truths are objective. Our moral disagreements become vehement, and can even lead to conflict, precisely when we believe that there is something really serious at stake – something that really matters, and matters enough that it requires us, and other people, to take action. In other words, what is at stake is something that we believe to be of objective significance for us all; we are simply not prepared to regard it as a matter of taste or individual preference, where subjective attitudes may legitimately differ, where standards may vary. Imagine that we discover a man who is busily skinning babies alive. He knows perfectly well what he is doing, and he does it for fun. And now imagine that someone – perhaps a very simple-minded person, or some sophisticated philosopher in the grip of a bizarre theory about morality – claims that we are mistaken in condemning this man as doing something that is objectively morally wrong. The man's actions – this person says – depart from *our* relative standards; but relative to *his own* standards, his actions are perfectly acceptable, and it is not for us to condemn him, or to take action against him, or even to disagree with him; we merely note the difference between our moral beliefs and his. I trust that we would regard this claim not merely as false, but as outrageously false. Skinning babies alive for fun is wrong *full stop*. It is objectively wrong. This is a moral truth that we are simply not prepared to regard as merely relative. And we regard it as such an important truth that we insist that consistent action is required. All of us are morally required to observe this truth, and where action to the contrary occurs – where someone *does* skin babies alive for fun – we are required to act instantly to intervene.

And there are many other moral truths that we regard in the same way. We take them to be objective truths; we are simply not prepared to treat them as merely relative. For instance, Hitler's policies were wrong. The appalling genocides of recent decades have been wrong. And so on. But we don't need to look only to those spectacular acts of wickedness on the global scale, or to something as unthinkable as the skinning of live babies, to note policies and actions which all of us can recognise as deserving our clear condemnation. We can look much closer to home, for the caring professions themselves offer many examples. Consider the following kinds of case.

As we noted in Chapter One, over recent decades there has been a flowering of codes of ethics for health and other professions. One of the most important of these modern codes is the World Medical Association's Declaration of Geneva, first adopted in 1948. The global medical profession was particularly moved to formulate this code when it became aware of what some of its members had been involved in during the Second World War. A considerable number of doctors in Germany and Japan had taken part in serious, well-organised programmes of experimentation upon, and elimination of, persons under their care. Concentration camp inmates and other prisoners were used as guinea pigs in unspeakably cruel experiments. And within a so-called euthanasia programme, an enormous number of patients who suffered from some medical problem or disability were killed because they were regarded as unfit – as "useless eaters", or "life unworthy of life", as the Nazis described them. The medical doctors were devoting their professional skill, in other words, to programmes of torture and mass murder. (A few of these doctors were tried at Nuremberg after the war.)

In January 2000, Dr Harold Shipman, an English general practitioner, was convicted of the murder of 15 of his patients. A subsequent judicial inquiry estimated that over a 27-year period, Shipman had in fact murdered 250 of his patients. His typical method was to administer a lethal dose of morphine, and to falsify the death certificate and his own medical records in order to claim that the patient had been in poor health. Most of his victims were elderly women, and most had in fact been in good health. In January 2004 Shipman committed suicide in prison, without having confessed to or explained his crimes.

A gynaecologist commits a series of sexual assaults upon his patients while performing clinical examinations, and afterwards threatens that he will claim that they implored his sexual favours if they report what he has done.

A surgeon in a small country hospital performs a series of operations after enjoying drunken lunches at the local pub. A number of his patients are seriously harmed by his botched procedures.

A night nurse on duty, while reading her newspaper at the nurse's station, chooses to ignore the alarm from an elderly patient's room at 11.50pm. Day-shift nurses, on their rounds the next morning, discover this patient dead on the floor of her room. She had fallen during the night and managed to crawl to reach the alarm button.

A man brutally murders his wife and baby. During the preceding months, the social worker to whom that family had been assigned for case management had turned a blind eye to repeated evidence of serious domestic violence.

A clinical psychologist wilfully manipulates a small child's drawings, using the results as the basis of an accusation (which is otherwise completely unsupported, and in fact false) that the child's father has been sexually abusing the child.

And we could cite, or imagine, many other such cases. They are all cases in which a member of the caring professions has done something wrong. Perhaps we will wish to say that some of those offences are *more* wrong than others: some involve neglect or indifference or recklessness, whereas others are horrifyingly intentional. But in each case the wrong is clear, and it is a wrong that we can all recognise as worthy of moral condemnation. And suppose, once again, that someone protests against this, claiming that what we are condemning is wrong only relative to *our* standards, and that there are alternative moral standards by which that behaviour is *not* wrong: "Nazi morality is just *different* from our morality. What the Nazi doctors did was right by their standards, and it's not for us to impose our standards upon them…" We would surely respond by rejecting this protest as utterly unacceptable. The wrongs we observe in these cases are wrongs which we are simply not prepared to regard as merely relative.

I noted earlier that, in asking whether morality is objective, it might be difficult to produce as evidence some moral truths that we can all recognise as objective. But in fact, this turns out to be much less difficult than it may have seemed. For we have just been exposing a series of moral truths which we do recognise as objective. It is wrong to skin babies alive for fun. It is wrong to imprison innocent and vulnerable persons and use them as mere guinea pigs in horrifically cruel experiments. It is wrong to commit rape. It is wrong to neglect the needs of persons whose care is our responsibility. It is wrong to bring a false accusation against someone. And so on. We can recognise those clear moral truths simply by stating what we have observed about the cases we have just noted. And we can also see that those rather particular and specific moral truths are nested within a series of more general moral truths which we can all recognise. For instance, it is wrong to commit murder. It is wrong to steal. We ought to respect one another and one another's rights. We ought to behave honestly towards one another. We ought to keep our promises. We ought to act justly and fairly. Love is good. Selfishness, meanness, callousness and cruelty are bad. And so on and so on… Now it is true that some of the items on that list are principles to which we believe there are morally legitimate exceptions. Those principles are more like general rules of thumb than absolutely strict rules. (We will discuss this later.) But all the same, we regard such claims as those on that list as objectively correct. We are not prepared to regard them as merely relatively true – true merely for us. Indeed, as we noted earlier, we find that such truths and principles are in fact very commonly recognised by different people across different cultures, and we even see such principles appealed to when people try to offer excuses for wicked behaviour. And it is because we regard such principles as binding upon us all that we believe action is required when they are seriously violated – even, if necessary, violent action.

Of course, we should further note that those principles guide us not only in our condemnations of what is morally wrong, but also in our praise of what is morally commendable. Those doctors and nurses and social workers, for instance, who tirelessly devote themselves to the care of their needy patients or clients, receiving little reward, and often at great cost to themselves, are doing something morally splendid. And this, too, is an evaluation which we are not prepared to regard as merely relative. Somebody might say, "Well, *you* regard that kind of conduct as splendid; but this verdict of yours is no more legitimate than the view that the Nazi doctors, devoting themselves to their experimenting and killing, were engaged in morally splendid conduct." But again, we would reject this as utterly unacceptable.

Let us review the ground we have covered in this chapter so far. We have been responding to an objection to the very study of ethics. The objection arises from the worry that there is no objective subject matter to be studied. The worry is that morality is merely relative – to different people and different cultures. We can compare different moral standards, but we can't presume to announce, or to apply, objectively correct standards which are true for us all, for there are no such things. And our response to that worry has been in two parts. First, we critically assessed the argument used to support moral relativism. We saw that this argument is invalid: for even if it were true that different people or cultures have different moral views, it need not be true that there is no such thing as objective moral truth. And we noted that in any case, the premise of this argument is false; for, at least at the level of deep moral principles, different people and cultures in fact share many of the same moral views. Secondly, we tackled relativism head-on by noting various ways in which we are certainly committed to the objectivity of morality. We believe in moral progress and regress. We believe in real moral disagreement. And there are many moral judgements which we are simply not prepared to regard as merely relatively true. And these judgements arise from general moral principles which we take to be objectively correct – the principles, in fact, which we find to be shared by different peoples and different cultures, and which are recognised even by those who seek to offer excuses for immoral behaviour, and to which we appeal when we condemn some behaviour as immoral or praise it as morally splendid.

The clash between different world-views

Nevertheless, we have not yet addressed every part of the worry that ethics cannot be an objective study. When we heard that worry expressed, it was pointed out that there are, in particular, serious differences between the moral views of so-called religious people, on the one hand, and non-religious people, on the other. We can readily think of such differences in views on particular ethical topics – on questions, for instance, concerning the beginning of life, such as abortion; and concerning the ending of life, such as euthanasia; and concerning sexual behaviour and sexual identity; and so on. But there are also differences concerning *how* we ought to reach our moral conclusions: many religious people will insist that we cannot get the right answers without paying attention to the commands and purposes of God; whereas so-called non-religious people will, of course, reject that view. Those various differences run deep: they proceed from very different fundamental beliefs, and the people who hold those beliefs are deeply *committed* to their positions. It is foolish to think that people will readily give up their most basic beliefs, which form their whole view of the world, and indeed their very identity. So how can it *not* be foolish to think that they will be able to sit down with people operating from quite different world-views and reason together towards shared moral conclusions? Don't we have good reason, then, to doubt that an objective reasoned enquiry into ethics, in which people with quite different world-views can all equally take part, is even possible?

Now there is a serious point expressed here, which I do not think we can dodge. We need to consider it directly. And to do this, we need to think for a little while about the relation between moral views and so-called religious or non-religious commitments.

We could spend a lot longer than a little while in considering whether something should be called a religion, and then in reviewing the vast variety of different beliefs which might be described as religious, as well as those which might be described as non-religious or anti-religious. But important as those questions are, I do not want us to get bogged down by them here. For I think that, for our purposes here, we can usefully simplify the discussion by concentrating on the contrast between the two world-views which are most prominent in contemporary ethical debates, at least in the Western world. On the one hand, there is the world-view often called naturalism. This is the view that the natural world, which includes us human beings, is all that exists. There is nothing that transcends the natural world. There is no god; there are no purposes other than our own purposes; and so on. I will refer to someone who holds this view as an atheist. On the other hand, there is the view shared by people whose beliefs are grounded in the Judaeo-Christian tradition. They believe in the God described in the biblical scriptures, and in God's purposes and commands there described, and so on. Of course, people within this tradition can differ from one another in many of their beliefs; but for our purposes, I am largely ignoring those differences and concentrating on the general picture presented by this world-view. Though in describing the content of this world-view, I am going to focus on Christian beliefs – partly because the Christian narrative has exercised an especially weighty influence on Western ethical thought, not least in the caring professions, and because it provides the starkest contrast with the naturalistic picture.[2] I will refer to someone who holds this general view as a theist.[3] And for simplicity's sake, let us imagine that these two views represent the full range of world-views which need to be taken into account. As we shall note below, the moral consequences of these two world-views offer us a very vivid contrast. (Naturalism differs far less from some Eastern religions, for instance, than it differs from what I have just labelled as theism.)

Of course, if we do imagine that these are the only possible views, the really vital question is which view is *true*. But I am not going to offer a case in answer to that question here (though I will reconsider it later on). It is a question which expresses an enormous and very live issue within the contemporary intellectual world, and on each side of the debate there are numerous very able philosophers (not to mention other people). But then, if we are not going to decide between these world-views, how can we hope to proceed to common ethical discussion?

There is an argument which is commonly used to try to persuade us that we can break out of the impasse and make progress here. It is an argument to the effect that we can in fact *ignore* one of those opposing world-views. The argument is favoured particularly by philosophers of an atheistic persuasion, and it seeks to show that we can *dismiss* theistic belief from our ethical discussions, not because we have shown that theism is *false*, but because we can show that it is, in a sense, *irrelevant*. It is an argument which goes back to Plato, and it proceeds by posing a dilemma for the theist – often referred to as the Euthyphro Dilemma, from the title of the dialogue in which Plato presents the argument. The argument starts by observing that theists typically want to connect our moral obligations, what we ought to do, with what God commands. But then it asks a question: is something obligatory (what we ought to do) because God commands it, or does God command it because it is what we ought to do? If the theist chooses the first of those alternatives, he or she is committed to saying that anything that God commands would thereby become obligatory. But this would mean that if, for instance, God commanded us to torture babies, then torturing babies would become something we ought to do. And this would surely be an untenable view. But if we choose the second alternative – that God commands something because it is something we ought to do – then it is not God's command that *makes* it something we ought to do. The obligation, what we ought to do, would be *independent* of God's command. But if obligations are independent of God's commands, then, in working out what our obligations are, we ought not to ask simply what God commands, for the fact that God commands something is no guarantee that it is what we ought to do. We would need to ask whether what is commanded *is* in fact what we ought to do. And if we *should* ask this, then of course we *can* enquire into our obligations without any reference to God's commands at all. (A similar question can be posed in response to the theist's typical connecting of moral goodness with God's will and purposes. Is something good because it is what God wills, or intends; or does God will it because it is good? The first alternative implies that anything willed by God would thereby be good, and therefore that, for instance, hatred and cruelty and unbearable suffering would be good if willed by God. But the second alternative implies that goodness is independent of what God wills; and in that case we can and should enquire into what goodness is without any reference to God's will.) The question posed by the argument is intended as a *dilemma* for the theist. It offers two, and only these two, possible answers. And the problem for the theist is that each answer may seem deeply unwelcome. One answer makes God's commands and will completely arbitrary, with the consequence that we might be morally obliged to do what seems to be morally unthinkable (torture babies, if that is what God commands). But the other answer severs the direct connection between morality and God (for moral requirements are then independent of God's commands). If theists choose the first answer, their position can be ignored, for they have thereby declared that they are prepared, in the name of obedience to God, to do the morally unthinkable; and why should that voice be heard in any serious and proper moral discussion? But if they choose the second answer, they have accepted that we cannot reach proper moral conclusions simply by asking what God commands or wills, and so they have accepted that we can pursue our ethical enquiries without any reference to God. Either way, we can ignore theism and get on with the business of reasoned ethical enquiry in just the way in which the atheist does get on with it. Or so the argument goes.

I imagine that the Euthyphro Dilemma would have been felt to carry particular bite within the ancient Greek world within which Plato posed it. For any cursory glance at the myths concerning the Graeco-Roman gods indicates that they were characters who were capable of all sorts of morally dubious shenanigans. There would indeed have been no guarantee that commands issued by them expressed genuine moral obligations.

However, the theist – adhering to the Judaeo-Christian tradition – will insist that it is impossible that God (the God of that tradition) would issue a command to torture babies, or indeed to do anything else that is wrong. For God is believed by the theist to be utterly good, and God's goodness is believed to be a core feature of who he is. (As the philosophers would put it, God is, according to the theistic conception, *essentially* good. He cannot fail to be good, and any being who is not completely good cannot be God.) So – the theist will claim – we can dismiss the possibility that God commands something immoral, or that God intends something bad. He is not an arbitrary tyrant. The Hebrew scriptures declare again and again that God, unlike the idolatrous gods of the surrounding nations, is holy and completely good, and that his commands and judgements are righteous. People are invited to "taste and see" that God is good, and to recognise the rightness and correctness of his commands. The clearly visible moral beauty and truth of God and his commands are repeatedly declared.

But now, this concedes at least part of Plato's point. For it shows that the theist, if he or she wishes to stand by these declarations, cannot also draw the simplest kind of equation between goodness and what God wills, or between moral rightness and what God commands. If to say that something is right *simply means* that it is what God commands, then to claim that God commands what is right is to claim that God commands what God commands, and this is utterly trivial. And if to say that something is good *simply means* that it is the way God wills, then to claim that God is good is to claim that God is the way God wills, which may be true but is morally completely uninformative.

But theists do not want to make merely trivial claims in saying that God is good and his commands are right. They want to be conveying what they in fact regard as vitally important *information*. What the theistic scriptures say is repeatedly declared as, to put it mildly, interesting and important *news* about God and his commands – news which cannot be expressed as a series of trivial and uninformative remarks.

So the information the theist wishes to convey concerning the goodness of God and the rightness of his commands would be prevented by drawing a simplistic equation – which some theists are, inconsistently, inclined to draw – between goodness and rightness and what God wills and commands. And such a simplistic equation would undermine the Hebrew *message* to the peoples of the world that they should *look* and *see* the goodness of God and the rightness of his commands (in contrast to the character and commands of other idolatrous gods).

But then, don't the theists have to accept the second horn of the Euthyphro Dilemma? They must concede that rightness doesn't simply mean what God wills. They claim that God is really good and his commands are really right. But in claiming this, they are in effect claiming that God's character and commands measure up to an independent set of moral standards – a set of standards against which that character and those commands can be assessed. Indeed, the theist has claimed that this is something that we can *recognise* – something that we can look at and *see*. The repeated Hebrew message takes for granted that people in general – the surrounding nations – do have enough knowledge of goodness and rightness to be able to recognise the real goodness of God and the real rightness of his commands. It takes for granted that people in general *can perform* their own evaluation of God's character and commands – weighing them against the independent moral standards by which they can be assessed. But if people in general can do this, then they possess real moral knowledge, and they do not need to resort to what God commands in order to put that knowledge to work. So isn't the theist obliged to concede the atheist's point? We don't need to refer to God at all in our ethical enquiries. And given that any claims about God are controversial, to say the least, we should ban talk of God from our ethical deliberations, and proceed on the basis of our common moral knowledge.

That, however, would be too swift a conclusion. Just as the theist can draw too simplistic a connection between morality and God, the atheist can too simplistically dismiss the connection. For what the theist believes entails that there is still a very important connection between God and morality. If theism is true, we should take the commands and purposes of God very seriously indeed. And this is so for a number of reasons.

First, if theism is true, then God is the moral authority *par excellence*. He will have a perfect knowledge of what is good and right. And this is not only because he is, according to the theist, omniscient – that is, all-knowing. It is also because he is omnipotent – that is, all-powerful – and completely good. According to the theist, everything in the world is due to and subject to God's power; so God is the creator and sustainer of everything. And because God is also completely good, the purposes for which he has created things are good purposes. And they are, of course, purposes which he knows. So he is in a unique position to say *what is best* for each created thing. Knowing how he has made each thing, and knowing how it fulfils its good purposes, God is uniquely able to say, with complete accuracy, how it will *flourish*. And this, of course, entails that if we wish to act for *the good* of those things that we affect by our actions, including ourselves, we will have no better guide than what God says. Whereas if we choose to ignore what God says, we are acting with *indifference* towards the good of the things we affect; and if we choose to act in a way that is contrary to what God says, then we are acting in a way that is *contrary to the good* of those things. So our moral duty to act for the good of the things we affect, including ourselves, and not to do evil to them, would be guided with complete accuracy by what God says. All this will be true if theism is true.

We saw that it is simplistic for the theist to claim that "right" just means "what God commands" and "good" just means "what God wills". But the theist believes that God is *essentially* good; so if theism is true, it will be the case that whatever God wills is in fact good, and whatever he commands is in fact right. And what we have now noted about God's purposes in creating things shows that there *is*, after all, a sense in which God's will *brings it about* that we have various moral duties. For (if theism is true) it is because of God's will that something is created as it is, with the nature it has, and it is because it has this nature that it will flourish under the conditions in which it does flourish. (It is because of its nature that a seed flourishes while buried in soil. It is because of its nature that a human being does not flourish while buried in soil…) So it is God's will that makes it true that it is *best* for that thing to be treated in certain ways – the ways that allow it to flourish. And so it is God's will that makes it true that we have particular moral duties towards that thing – those particular duties to act in the ways that are for its good, and to avoid acting in ways that would do evil to it. Thus, for instance, it is because of God's will in creating human beings as they are that we have a particular duty not to bury other living humans in soil. (Of course, this is not to say that we have a moral duty to ensure that *everything* flourishes. We need not have the same duty towards the seed as towards the human being, and this difference between duties could be due to a number of factors. For instance, the flourishing of the seed might, because it grows into a poisonous plant, pose a risk to the flourishing of the human. Or the flourishing of this particularly vigorous plant species might pose a risk to other plant species. And so on. But the proper flourishing of things in their relations to each other will depend upon the natures that God has given to those various things – natures that are due to God's will.) To know how to do good to things, and to avoid doing evil to them, we need to know the conditions under which they will flourish, in their relations to other things. Those conditions are dependent upon the purposes with which God has created those things. And so those conditions could not be better understood than by listening to God's statement of his purposes.

So God is uniquely positioned to inform us, with complete accuracy, how to act to do good and avoid evil in relation to everything, including ourselves. I say that God's information would be completely *accurate*. But I do not think that the theistic story entails that the information would be *complete*. For it is a feature of the story that humans are given a very great significance, and this significance includes a considerable responsibility for our own flourishing, and for the care of others and the world. Nor is this a merely static significance, for we can choose to learn how to *extend* the caring difference we can make for ourselves and others and the world. But in order to be able to learn this, we need to be given the responsibility to *find out* many facts about how to do good and avoid evil. (And in this respect the story of course accords with our common-sense experience, for we spend a good deal of our time and effort in discovering the natures of things and the conditions under which they flourish.) But if God *does* provide information – in his commands about how we are to act, and in the descriptions of his purposes for things – then this is presumably because it is particularly important information that we need to hear for the purposes of responsible action, and so we would, to say the least, be foolish to ignore it.

And we can imagine various ways in which the moral clarity we would gain from such information would be especially helpful. We may be uncertain or even mistaken about how to act simply because the morally correct course is unclear. The situation in which we have to decide how to act may be complicated and confusing – perhaps because it is difficult to identify exactly what *would* be good for ourselves or others. Or perhaps we are liable to moral error not so much because the moral course is difficult to discern as because our own ability to discern that course has been compromised. We may be mistaken about how to act in the best interests of ourselves and others because we have absorbed errors concerning the conditions under which we truly flourish: our sense of what is best might have been perverted by constant familiarity with a lower standard. In these sorts of cases the information provided by God may give us the clarity we need.

Or perhaps we are ourselves wilfully responsible for the corruption of our moral discernment. Earlier in this chapter we noted that there is plenty of behaviour in the world around us which we readily condemn as immoral. And we noted that people typically seek to offer excuses for their immoral behaviour. Now those excuses are often the product of rationalisation and self-deception. ("This is not the theft of another nation's territory; it is the righteous liberation of folk who properly belong to the fatherland…" "We are not eliminating true human beings; we are purging the nation of a sub-human source of deadly infection…" Or perhaps closer to home: "I might not have done the work, but I was the real brains behind the idea, so only my name ought to be on the poster…" "The company of course *wants* us to be able to work outside office hours, so there's no problem in my taking this untagged computer home…" "I am already so heavily taxed that it would be unjust for me to have to declare what is in any case this trivial amount of further income…" "I am merely offering this woman some of the tender loving care she clearly deserves; I am not threatening her marriage. Anyway, if her marriage *is* threatened by genuine love, then it's not a marriage worth hanging on to…" "The man in need on the other side of the road is not my responsibility. And I would simply be complicating the situation unhelpfully by getting involved. And in any case the appointment I'm heading to is especially important…" And so on.) Humans have a remarkable ability to deceive themselves about their own motivations and intentions, and to convince themselves that their wrong actions are in fact morally justified. (And this is no doubt one of the reasons why we recognise immorality much more clearly in other persons than in ourselves, for we have hidden from ourselves our own immoral attitudes and intentions, or we have cloaked them in the rationalisations which allow us to believe that we have nothing to be ashamed of.) And from this obvious fact about human nature, it follows that we do not always approach moral decisions with entirely clear, uncluttered minds, and wills directed towards what is right and good. Our wills can be compromised by morally unsatisfactory motivations (our laziness and desire not to make an uncomfortable effort; our greed; our various lusts, including our lust for power, or for self-aggrandisement; and so on, and so on), and our minds can be compromised by the rationalisations and deceptions we have allowed ourselves to accept. But God's commands, as we have noted, will be completely uncompromised: they will state the requirements of perfect, holy goodness. And thus they may bring into the darkness and confusion of our own moral deliberations the very light we require for moral clarity. Clear commands which come not from ourselves, but from a perfect moral authority might expose our rationalisations and self-deceptions for what they are.

That, then, is one respect in which, according to the theist, there is a very important connection between God and morality. The theist will insist that information we receive about the commands and purposes of God will provide *moral guidance* which we should take very seriously.

But that is not the only important connection which the theist draws between God and morality. For the theist can also insist that what we learn about the commands and purposes of God can *move* us to take our moral duties properly seriously. If theism is true, our moral duties are to be accompanied by especially serious concern, even worry; but also by serious hope. What do I mean by this?

If we are going to be *motivated* to act in morally proper ways, it helps if we know that we are *accountable* for our behaviour. But to what extent are we *actually* accountable? We are, of course, accountable to our fellow human beings. We can be praised by them for our morally worthy conduct and held to account for our immoral conduct – *but* only to the extent that these other persons are *aware* of what we do. If we can manage to get away with immoral behaviour, then we will not be held accountable by them. And if they happen to share in our immoral behaviour or attitudes, then we will no doubt receive their approval or acquiescence where we deserve blame, and this accountability will be morally worthless. We are also accountable to ourselves: our own consciences can call us to account. But as we have just been pointing out, our own consciences can be compromised by our rationalisations and self-deceptions, and thus we can all too readily content ourselves with behaviour of which we ought to be ashamed. So if the atheistic picture is correct, then moral accountability is a very imperfect business. However, if theism is true, then there is real moral accountability – accountability which is both perfect and inescapable. If God exists, he is aware of everything about our intentions and actions. He assesses them by completely uncompromised, perfect standards. And in the final analysis, he calls us all to account. If the fact that we are accountable can serve to motivate us towards morally satisfactory behaviour, then on the theistic picture, we have seriously powerful motivation to behave as we ought to behave.

According to the great German philosopher Immanuel Kant, our behaviour ought to be motivated *simply and entirely* by our seeking to do our moral duty. In particular, we ought not to be motivated by thoughts of reward or punishment. For if we were seeking some reward or the avoidance of punishment, then we would be motivated by our own self-interest, and this would not be a properly *moral* motivation. Truly moral motivation seeks to do what is right simply *because* it is right. And no doubt Kant is making an important point here. But *are we* in fact motivated as we ought to be? We have already pointed out the unhappy answer to this question. Our wills can be seriously compromised by morally unsatisfactory motivations – by those desires which move us to act in directions contrary to our moral duty, and which prompt the lies we tell ourselves in rationalising our immoral behaviour. And these rationalisations may provide us with some sense of moral comfort if we are called to account by nothing more exacting than our own compromised conscience and the judgements of our similarly unsatisfactory fellow human beings. However, if we know that we are called to account by a morally perfect judge, who sees everything not only about our actions, but also about our desires and attitudes and intentions and the stories we tell ourselves, then this may provide just the spur we need to put our motivations in order. Just as an awareness of God's clear commands might expose our self-deceptions, awareness of our accountability to God can motivate us in the direction in which Kant says that we ought to be motivated – to do what is right.

Even so, the idea of being morally accountable to a perfect God is – at least for most of us – a seriously worrying prospect. (This can surely fuel a temptation to relieve ourselves of the worry by ridding ourselves of the thought that it could be true.) And the fact that we find the prospect worrying is quite sufficient in itself to indicate to us our own moral condition, for there would be nothing worrying about the thought of being accountable to God if we were morally satisfactory persons. However, I said that on the theistic picture, our moral duties are accompanied not only by worry but also by hope. And this is because the picture entails that we can be *helped* towards morally proper behaviour – helped not only to *do* what is right, but to *want* and to *will* to do what is right. This hope comes from the rest of the theistic narrative. For the theistic story is an account not only of God's moral perfection, but also of his incalculably generous love. It is a story not just of judgement, but also of redemption. And the redemption it describes includes our being forgiven for our moral failures and assisted by God to act in ways that we cannot reliably achieve for ourselves. It includes the offer of power that can bring about a moral transformation of our human nature – a transformation even of our natural inclinations, and a new wisdom to discern what is right. The story offers the prospect of our becoming morally satisfactory persons – indeed, wonderfully admirable persons. And this would surely add serious weight to our moral motivation. If we can be forgiven for our failures and given help to improve, then our seeking to live a moral life is not a hopeless task, and we have excellent reason to persevere. Furthermore, our behaviour would be motivated not merely by a concern to fulfil moral requirements, but also by a glad and grateful submission to the God who rules the whole universe, who gives us our very existence, and who is extending to us his gift of redemption. The love that he extends to us would prompt our thankful love in return. And we would be moved also to extend our own love towards other persons who are loved by God, and to extend our care towards the rest of God's creation. Our transformation would thus include our becoming *people of love – motivated* by love. This change in us as we submit to the transforming power of God would no doubt be slow and gradual, even painful; but according to the theistic narrative, it is genuine. And we would have every incentive to submit to this change because it would help us not only to understand and to do what is right, but also to enjoy what is best for ourselves. For our own real flourishing, our true happiness, would consist in undergoing this redemptive transformation. Here the love of God, the love of others, and the love of ourselves all come together. For of course, there is nothing objectionable in wanting what is best for ourselves if that is exactly what enables us to want and to do the best for everyone else.

The theist could add much more to this picture, which I have described in the barest, most summary terms. But even this simple sketch is enough to display some of the distinctive features of the theistic world-view – features not shared by the naturalistic picture held by the atheist, but features which are certainly relevant to morality. We see that there are very significant differences between the theistic picture and the naturalistic picture with respect to our knowing *what* to do and our being moved and enabled to *do* it. The theist will feel that we are foolish to ignore those features. He or she will feel that we cannot engage in adequately informed ethical enquiry if we leave those features out of the discussion. Whereas the atheist will, of course, feel that none of those distinctive features has any proper place within our ethical discussion because they are not features of the true state of affairs.

How, then, are we to proceed with our ethical enquiry while those different points of view stare us in the face? We might try to resolve this problem by *adjudicating* between those different world-views – by trying to discover which of them is true (even assuming, of course, that there are no other world-views that need to be considered). But as I said before, I shall not attempt that very substantial task here. But if we cannot decide between the different views, what are we to do? Many philosophers proceed by simply *presuming* that one of those views is false, but to any critical observer this looks like a mere unjustified prejudice – and, of course, it alienates those who don't start out with the conviction that the dismissed world-view is false. But how, then, are we to proceed?

A way to move forward

Given all that I have said, it may come as a surprise that I propose to proceed *largely* in the way that the atheist would want to proceed. In the next two chapters – in the remainder of Part A of this book – I shall seek to pursue our ethical enquiry without making any reference to God or his commands and purposes. I shall seek to appeal only to the kinds of considerations which the atheist might endorse. But how can this strategy be justified? Well, let us look at it from the perspective of each of the conflicting world-views, in turn.

The atheists will obviously approve of my proposed strategy. It is the strategy which they would pursue themselves. They believe that the theistic story is fiction and that its distinctive features ought therefore to be ignored, as having no relevance to a real moral conversation in which we are guided by the truth.

But interestingly enough, the theists can also approve of this strategy – at least to a considerable extent. And their reasons for doing so have already been suggested by our review of their narrative. For as we saw, they claim that ordinary people can recognise the goodness of God and the rightness of his commands and purposes. But it would not be possible for ordinary people to do this unless they possessed enough moral knowledge for real moral discernment – the knowledge required to recognise what is real goodness and rightness, and to distinguish it from what is not. In other words, the theists' claim takes for granted that people in general can operate with a moral sense which does not depend upon a prior knowledge of God's commands and purposes. (Theists believe that this moral sense – like our ability to grasp truths concerning the natural world, and like everything else we possess – *comes from* God, even if we don't recognise that it does.) And this theme runs through the rest of the theistic narrative. In many ways, the narrative either asserts or takes for granted that those who do not believe in God can exercise moral discernment and judgement, and identify and commend real goodness. On the theistic picture, we have an implicit sense of many of God's commands and purposes. We are equipped with the sense we require to be able to recognise, or to discover, what is best for each created thing, so that we can care for it and allow it to flourish. And in particular, the narrative asserts that we are *all* accountable to God for the conduct of our lives because we can all tell the difference between right and wrong.[4] And this theistic theme is, of course, consistent with what we observed earlier of the common moral sense possessed by different people and different cultures.

So the two contrasting world-views converge in this respect. Each of those different viewpoints offers reason to believe that ordinary people everywhere can operate with a reliable moral sense. And this provides the basis for the way I wish to proceed in our subsequent discussion. I propose to pursue our ethical enquiry by appealing only to what people in general might be expected to endorse – whatever else they believe, and whether or not they believe in God.

I said that this is *largely* the way in which the atheist would proceed. In the next two chapters (the remainder of Part A of the book), where we concentrate on setting out ethical basics, I shall particularly try to appeal only to a general moral sense. But even here, we need to be on the lookout for ways in which the different world-views would lead us towards different moral judgements. If such differences arise, we would be proceeding unrealistically if we were to ignore them. And there may be places in which the theist believes that more needs to be said – a more that emerges from the distinctive features of the theistic narrative. If so, this will need to be noted. We can think of our discussion in this part of the book as a kind of *experiment*, testing the idea that we can gather common ethical foundations for shared moral conclusions.

However, in Part B of the book – where we come to some longer case studies, applying the basics gathered in Part A – we will find that the dependence on common ground comes under greater strain. There we will do what we can to work towards conclusions which we can all accept; but we will find, I think, that world-view differences become significant and unable to be ignored. And we will need to think about how to respond to those differences.

It seems to me, then, that we can proceed with cautious confidence. Our response to the challenge of relativism indicates that we can have some confidence that there is enough common moral sense for us to reason together within an objective ethical enquiry. But this confidence needs to be cautious and careful. We ought not to be naïve in expecting our discussion to be thoroughly enlightened. Our moral sense can be confused or perverted. Our world-view beliefs may lead us in different directions. We need to reflect critically upon the arguments and judgements we hear from others, but also upon those we are ourselves inclined to offer.

For there is a big difference between confidence and arrogance. If relativism is false – if there is a real, objective difference between right and wrong – then moral judgements can be incorrect. And that includes our own judgements, not just those of others. We need to proceed humbly and diligently in the light of that sobering possibility. For in ethical enquiry, we are dealing with the most important matters – the matters that matter most.

Notes

1 There are contexts in which we talk of someone having *good* or *bad* taste. And in talking in that way, we are taking for granted that there is an objective standard against which the person's taste can be measured. But for the purposes of our discussion here, I am ignoring those kinds of case.

2 Christians believe that their narrative completes the narrative otherwise shared by the Abrahamic faiths. As we shall note, the distinctive Christian beliefs concerning redemption describe particular moral resources which are much less clearly entailed, if entailed at all, by the beliefs of non-Christian Jews and Muslims; and those particular resources provide further particular contrast with the naturalistic moral picture.

3 Because I am including specifically Christian beliefs within what I am calling the theistic narrative, I am here using the word "theist" in a particular, narrow sense. I do this simply to have an easy label for the narrative I am here referring to. This particular sense of the word should not be confused with the wider sense it has in general philosophical discussion. Readers who are familiar with the standard philosophical sense of the word should interpret my use of the word "theism" as denoting Christian theism.

4 Theists who are inclined to doubt this might read Chapter 2 of Paul's *Epistle to the Romans*. The theme has been elaborated in a variety of ways by different Christian theologians over the centuries.

4
Philosophical theories and professional ethics

We have discussed the common moral sense which enables us to make shared moral judgements, and we have noted various examples of those judgements. But can we say more about the basis of moral judgements? How do they come about? How should they come about? What general principles can guide us towards correct moral judgements? What is it about something that makes it right or wrong, good or bad?

Philosophers have in fact said much more in answer to those and related questions. They have offered a variety of theories concerning how our moral judgements arise, how they ought to be formed, and how they ought to be assessed. It can be important for professionals to have some working understanding of what the philosophers have said here, for the philosophical theories are certainly influential in the discussions of professional ethical questions. But it is a mixed bag of influences. Some of the philosophical theories offer insight and illumination which can be very helpful in professional ethics. Others can lead us dangerously astray. I think that every philosopher would agree with what I have just said in the last three sentences. They simply disagree about *which* theories are helpful and which are dangerous. For we are in contentious territory here.

I propose in this chapter to review some of the main features of this disputed philosophical terrain, and to point to places where I believe we can gain genuinely helpful insight, and to other places where danger lies. My views, though quite common, will be controversial; so – as everywhere else in this book – my readers need to be asking whether I am offering a sound basis for my assessments. I want my readers to be exercising their own critical skills, but not only in considering what *I* say. For, more generally and importantly, they need to be able to identify and critically evaluate the influences of the various philosophical theories upon the voices to be heard within their own unfolding professional ethical discussions; and I hope that this chapter will help towards that end.

DOI: 10.4324/9781003176541-5

Egoism

It is useful to begin by considering the question of the origin of our moral rules. Where do they come from, and how are they brought about? Let's start by examining a particular kind of theory which offers what is essentially a simple answer to that question. Its key idea is *self-interest*, and so a theory of this kind is called an ***egoist*** theory. There are a number of versions of this kind of theory, but they typically involve a combination of the following elements.

First, there is the claim that each one of us is in fact motivated – solely, or at least largely – by our own self-interest. We seek to do and to gain what we ourselves want, what we consider best *for ourselves*. And we are *not* motivated – at all, or at least very much – by a concern *for others*. This claim, as a *description* of our human condition, is called ***psychological egoism***.

The next step is to argue that our common-sense moral rules, which do require us to act with a concern for others, arise as we consider the best way to gain what we want for ourselves. How does this work? Let's think about what life would be like if every one of us were to act very directly out of our own nakedly self-interested motivations. Your wishes would get in the way of mine, for there would be times and places at which we would want the very same thing. We would all be in competition, and this would lead to conflict. We would be motivated to win these competitions by whatever methods we could use to gain some advantage – including by killing, stealing, lying and deceiving. But unless my power and vigilance were greater than anyone else's, I would be in very serious danger of being killed and robbed myself. And as my lies were discovered, I would not be trusted, and I would be deceived in return. I would have no reason to believe what other people told me. I would be unable to rely upon other people or work co-operatively with them. And so I would be unable to achieve any of those things that cannot be achieved without information I need to get from other people, or without their co-operation and assistance. Our life in this natural state would be – to use the famous words of 17th Century English philosopher Thomas Hobbes – "solitary, poor, nasty, brutish, and short".[1] In other words, if we *were* to act simply as we self-interestedly wished to act, we would *not* achieve what we self-interestedly want, for our life would be horrible. But then how *can* we achieve what we do want? The answer given by Hobbes and his followers is this. If we were to think rationally about our situation, each of us would recognise that the best way to achieve the greatest amount of what we ourselves want is by behaving according to rules that we would all agree to observe. If you and I (and others) agree not to kill one another, then we will not pose a threat to each other's lives. If we agree not to steal, we will not pose a threat to each other's property. If we agree to tell the truth and to keep our promises and to co-operate in various ways, we will be able to achieve goals that we could not achieve on our own. And so on. (And if we set up appropriate social arrangements and instruments – if we devise a "social contract" – we can ensure that these rules are *enforced*.) In this way, then, my moral duties *towards others* arise simply from my only fundamental duty – my duty to *myself*. Hence, a theory of this kind is called ***ethical egoism***. The ethical egoist claims that fundamentally, the only thing we ought to do is pursue our own self-interest. But we can see that it is rational to obey the common moral rules because *by doing so* we best advance our own self-interest.

Many philosophers have been attracted by the naturalism of ethical egoism – that is, by the fact that it offers an account of morality entirely in terms of what can go on in the natural world. We don't need to suppose that there is any morality at the ground level, as it were. And nor do we need to suppose that morality is delivered to us from on high. We are merely animals, operating in pursuit of what we individually desire. But we are rational animals, who can recognise that what we individually desire is best achieved through co-operation, and therefore by following the rules which make co-operation possible. And thus morality comes into existence. The common moral rules are a kind of *construction* out of our own self-interest.

What should we think of this theory? It seems to me that the egoist is offering what is in many ways a shockingly realistic account of the natural human condition. Selfishness does seem to be the driving motivation of an enormous amount of human activity, and the cause of so very many of the evils we observe in the world – evils that could be put right if humans were to co-operate according to sensible rules. And it is surely true that life for most of us is already much better than it would be if we did not obey common moral rules at least to the extent that we do.

But does the egoist offer a *fully* adequate description of the human condition, and a fully adequate account of the derivation of morality? It seems to me that the answer to each of those questions is No.

Despite the prevalence of selfishness, there is surely also – at least in some people, at some times – a good deal of ***altruism***; of genuine concern for others. We observe ordinary people acting altruistically in countless ways – towards their family and friends; towards their neighbours; even towards other people with whom they are not acquainted. Some people perform actions that we describe as *selfless*. Many people *devote* their lives to the care of others; and occasionally, we even witness cases in which people *sacrifice* their lives for others. As an adequate description of the human behaviour we actually observe, psychological egoism appears to be false.

Now the psychological egoist will typically respond by claiming that these cases are merely *apparent* instances of altruism, and that they are *actually* to be explained as instances of egoism. When people act in these ways, he will say, they do so because they are trying to gain what they *most want*. They are doing what will make *them* feel good, or what they think will please God, or secure a heavenly reward. So they are acting in pursuit of what they most powerfully desire; and so they are acting fundamentally for *their own* benefit, after all.

But this response is surely mistaken in a number of ways. It does not square with what we actually observe, and it involves a number of confusions. We can unravel these confusions by thinking more carefully about the relations between what we *feel* and *want* and what we *do*.

First, it is true that we do sometimes act for the good of others because we straightforwardly *desire* to do so. The actions that spring from our natural affections and sympathies can be of this kind. But this does not mean that we are acting for our own sake rather than for the sake of the others. For we can *desire* to act *altruistically*; we can *want* to act *for the sake of the others*. The fact that I am doing something because I want to do it does not show that I am doing it for my own sake.

And anyway, it is often the case that when we act for the good of others, believing that we *ought* to act that way, we have to act *against* our most powerful desires. Acting for the sake of others is often *hard*, and it can *hurt* – precisely because it clashes with what we desire most. (Effort is difficult when we desire to rest; fasting is uncomfortable because we desire to eat; and so on. And acting for the good of another is hard when we desire instead to act for our own good.) So it is simply false to claim that we act for the good of others only because this is what we most powerfully desire, if by "desire" we are talking about something that we *feel*. When we act for someone else's good, we may be acting for that *purpose*, and this may well be our most important purpose at that time. But in acting for that purpose, we may be acting in a way that is *contrary* to our most powerful desires.

Now it is true that we sometimes talk of our purposes in terms of what we *want*. Sometimes we talk of our most important purposes, or commitments, as our deepest wants, or our deepest desires – perhaps as the desires of our heart. And some of us harbour, among our deepest purposes, the commitment to act as we believe that we *ought* to act – including the commitment to act for the good of others. In this case it will be true that, in this sense of "want", we want to act for the good of others. It may also be true that from time to time, we experience something like a *longing*, a deeply felt wish, to act as we believe we ought to act, including for the good of others. But again, this would be a wish to act *altruistically*. And again, we nevertheless find that our actual *acting* for the good of others often has to be done in the teeth of our *felt* desires. We often have to act in a way that clashes with what we feel.

It is also true that we may well experience a *feeling of satisfaction* when we do act for the good of others, whether our action springs from natural felt desires or from our deeper purposes. But this does not show that our action is merely motivated by self-interest. For the feeling of satisfaction may not be (and typically will not be) the *object*, or goal, of our action. When I pursue a course of action to build a house, I may feel great satisfaction when the building is completed. But this does not mean that the object of my course of action was the feeling of satisfaction. I did not pursue that course of action *in order to* feel the satisfaction. I pursued it in order to produce a house. The house was what I was aiming at; and once my purpose was achieved, I felt satisfaction as a consequence. Similarly, when acting for the good of others, my object is the good of the others. I am no more acting *in order* to feel satisfaction than I am acting with that motivation when I build a house. But satisfaction can be a happy consequence as well.

It is true, too, that we may believe that in acting for the good of others, we are *also*, in the long term and at the deepest level, acting in a way that is best *for ourselves*. For there are many wise voices through the ages who advise me that my own flourishing will come about most fully within a life that involves a real commitment to the flourishing of others. But again, this does not show that my actions for others are motivated merely by self-interest. If I am genuinely acting for the good of others, I am acting *for their sake* – whether or not I believe that this will in the end also be good for me. It is possible to love my neighbour while also loving myself.

So there can be a concern for the good of others alongside a concern for one's own good, plus the enjoyment of a sense of satisfaction once goods have been achieved. All these things can go together; and within this complex whole, there is real altruistic motivation and action.

Those wise voices who say that the life concerned for the good of others is the life best for me also advise me that I can be trained, and train myself, to act for the good of others; and that I can thereby develop *habits* to act in that way, and thereby make it *easier* for myself to act in that way. I can make acting for the good of others something that I more naturally *desire*. (We shall return to this theme when we talk about the virtues later in this chapter.) But again, this does not show that in acting for the good of others I am merely acting to advance my own interests. It shows, rather, that it can become more natural for me to act *altruistically*. I can increasingly *want* to act altruistically. Altruistic action can become easier and more natural for me, and thus it may become more like those actions which spring from the affections and sympathies that are already natural. (But the person growing in virtue still finds that much action for the sake of others clashes with his felt self-interested desires.)

So altruism can be real. And that means that psychological egoism is a crudely inadequate picture of the human condition.

Thus the egoist gets the facts wrong, as far as his description of humanity is concerned. But his account of morality is also wrong. For ethical egoism is an unsatisfactory theory of how our common moral rules are derived, as we can see in the following way. Egoism tells us that we should follow the common moral rules because by doing so we will advance our own self-interest. And no doubt this is often true. No doubt it will often be the case that if I kill or steal or lie, then I will suffer some consequence – vengeance or punishment or lack of co-operation – that is greatly to my own disadvantage. But this need not *always* be the case. There may be occasions when I can get what I want by killing or stealing or lying, *and get away with it*. And now let us think about what the egoist would say of *these* cases. Of the usual sort of case, he says that I should obey the common moral rules because it is to my own benefit to do so. But in these exceptional cases, where I can get away with breaking those rules and thereby get what I want without suffering any harmful consequences, it is no longer to my benefit to observe the rules. And the egoist tells me that what I ought to do is to pursue my own interests. So he must say that in these particular exceptional cases, I ought to break the common rules. I ought to get what I want by killing, or stealing, or lying – so long as I can get away with doing so. So, in cases of this kind, egoism confers its blessing upon the free-rider, the cheat, the deceiver, the thief, the murderer, and so on.

Those are courses of action which egoism endorses on the *individual* level. And it grants its approval to similar actions at the *communal* level. Egoism tells communities to relate to one another according to accepted rules in order to avoid the harms of conflict and to enjoy the benefits of co-operation. But what if I belong to a community that is considerably more powerful than a neighbouring community, and this neighbouring community possesses goods that I want, or can be used in ways from which I would benefit? My community has the power to take what it wants, and here it can do so without any harmful consequence. So again, egoism would say that this is what my community ought to do. And thus it can approve oppression, tyranny, slavery, genocide, and so on – so long as my community can get away with it. It must also approve our destruction of the environment where that is to our advantage. For if *we* can benefit from our exploitation of the environment, and the harmful effects of what we do will occur only after we have died out, then the people who will be harmed by the damage we cause will belong to future generations. But those future generations cannot benefit *us*, so we have no reason to act for *their* benefit. In relation to my generation, the future generations are like communities that are completely subject to *our* power; so we have, according to the egoist, no reason to act for their good, given that we can act for our own good with complete impunity as far as they are concerned.

And now let us ask a question which I dare to hope we need to pose only rhetorically. Do we believe that the egoist is saying the right thing about these cases? Do we agree with him that in these cases there is no moral requirement to do what the ordinary moral rules would prescribe? Or do we believe, instead, that those moral rules *do* still apply, and therefore that they are showing that what the egoist tells us is wrong? Do we believe that in those situations where I can get away with it, my murdering, stealing and so on would *still* be *morally wrong*; and that where communities can get away with it, their oppression, tyranny, genocide, destruction of the environment, and so on, would still be *morally wrong*? Surely we do believe that these would be terrible wrongs. But the egoist cannot account for *why* they are wrong. According to him, something is wrong when it is contrary to our self-interest. But these courses of action would *achieve* our own interests, so the egoist cannot explain why they are wrong. If, however, we believe that they *are* clearly wrong, and that they are wrong in violating our moral rules, then we believe that our moral rules have a force and a basis which is not supplied by self-interest. We believe that murder, theft, cheating, tyranny, enslavement, and so on are wrong even when, by pursuing these courses of action, we can achieve what we want and successfully get away with it. The moral rules apply in places where the egoist would say that they do not apply; so the egoist is failing to account for the rules. The moral rules appear to have a deeper and more general validity than the egoist can explain.

Furthermore, we can criticise the egoist by accusing him of not thinking seriously enough, or sensitively enough, about where he should travel from his own starting point. His key idea is self-interest. But let's think for a moment about what that means and what can follow from it. When I ought to act to pursue my own interests, it is because my interests give me a *reason* for acting. If I can see that something would be for my good, then this gives me a reason to seek to attain that good for myself – for the person for whom it would be good. And I can recognise, more or less accurately, what would be for my good, because I understand what I need and what matters to me. Now my deepest needs – what matters to me for life, and for human flourishing – arise because of the way I am constituted. (I need food, shelter, bodily health, human interaction, and so on, because I am the kind of creature that I am, made the way that I am.) But if I can recognise what I need and what matters to me, and I can recognise that *you* are constituted similarly to the way that I am constituted, then I can recognise that *your* needs and concerns will be like mine. And if my recognition of what would be for my good gives me a *reason* for acting for that good for myself, then my recognition of what would be for *your* good *also* gives me a *reason* for acting for that good *for you* – for the person for whom it would be good. In recognising that something would be good, I have a reason for acting for that good for the person for whom it would be good – whether that person is you or me.

Or think about it this way. Suppose that I choose to promote only my good, and not also yours. If this choice is to be *reasonable*, there must be some relevant difference between the two goods. But the fact that only one of the goods would be *for me* is a merely *arbitrary* difference, not a relevant difference. For if something's being good provides a reason for pursuing it, then it provides that reason *in each case*. Two goods are at stake here, not one; and if I am concerned with goods at all, what *reason* can I have to concern myself only with one?

So it is a minute logical step from recognising what would be for my good to recognising also what would be for your good. Likewise, it is a minute logical step from recognising that the one good gives me a reason for action to recognising that the other good also gives me a reason for action. And we need only take one further minute logical step to recognise that we have a reason to pursue the good for *anyone else*. For anyone constituted similarly to the way I am constituted will share with me relevantly similar needs and concerns; and if this provides the ground for the recognition of what is for the good in the one case (mine), it does the same in every other such case as well. So, quite generally, if my good gives me reason to act to pursue that good for the person for whom it would be a good, then anyone else's good gives me similar reason to act.

What we have just done is trace a simple path from the egoist's starting point. He stresses self-interest. He takes it for granted that we have reason to act for our own good. But what we have just seen is that, starting from that point, there is a very compelling line of reasoning to the conclusion that we have reason to act for the good of others as well. Recognising the importance of self-interest also allows us to recognise the need for altruism.

Now this does not mean that I can always recognise what is for your good as well as you can yourself. Nor does it mean that I am always entitled to *act* for your good, at least without your permission; for my doing so might breach your right not to be interfered with. Furthermore, it may be that there is no need for me to act for your good, because you are doing so yourself, or others are doing it for you (though in such a case I would still have reason not to interfere with what is for your good). It may be that it would be good for you *that* you act for your own good – perhaps because you have a proper responsibility to do so. And nor does any of this mean that I always have a *desire* to act for your good which is as powerful as my desire to act for my own good. But the point here is not a point about felt desires. It is a point about reason for action. Because I can recognise what is for my own good, and thereby have a reason for action, I can also – at least in many cases – recognise what is for your good, and thereby also have a reason for action. And where I do have a reason for action, it is *unreasonable* of me *not* to act in that way (unless there is another, overriding, reason to the contrary).

It is interesting to note that this connection between recognising and acting for our own interests, on the one hand, and recognising and acting for others' interests, on the other, is explicitly drawn by the biblical commandments which are presented as a summary of the moral requirements concerning our human relations: "Do unto others as you would have them do unto you"[2], and "Love your neighbour as yourself".[3]

In summary, then, egoism does offer some kernels of truth. It provides a useful reminder of how selfish we can be. And it correctly observes that human society would scarcely be possible at all unless we followed our moral rules at least a good deal of the time. However, egoism is unsatisfactory as a complete theory. It provides an inadequate description of human action, and an inadequate account of how our moral rules come about. And it is blind to the path of reason which leads from its own starting point to altruism.

But perhaps I do not need to belabour the inadequacies of egoism in a book on the ethics of the caring professions. For the whole point of these professions is not to advance our own interests, but *to care for others in need*. These professions take altruism for granted. And while I sincerely hope that the people who work in these professions *enjoy* their work and indeed gain immense *satisfaction* from their work, I am confident that they typically pursue their profession *because* they wish to care for those in need. I am confident, in other words, that their motivation is typically not the crudely self-interested motivation described by egoism.

So let us leave egoism and turn now to those philosophical theories which suppose, as our ordinary moral rules do suppose, that altruism has a real and central place in morality – which suppose, in other words, that a concern for others is not a mere construction out of, and in pursuit of, our own self-interest, but a genuine moral requirement of its own.

Consequentialism versus deontology

When we turn to theories of this kind, it is helpful to see them as offering different answers to a particular fundamental question. The question is this:

what is it about an action that makes that action right or wrong? It is useful to begin by comparing two of the different kinds of theory that offer answers to that question. One kind of theory holds that what makes an action right or wrong is *solely*, or *entirely*, a matter of what effects it brings about in the world – a matter of the action's *consequences*. According to this kind of theory – a ***consequentialist*** theory, as it is called – no action is right or wrong *in itself*; rather, it is right or wrong in virtue of its consequences. So, for instance, whether an act of killing would be right or wrong will depend on the consequences it would have if it were performed under its particular circumstances. (Typical consequences of the killing of some person would include, obviously, his removal from the world and thus the non-occurrence of what he would have experienced and done in the life which is taken; and the grief which his death would cause in others; and his absence from the lives of those near and dear to him; and the need for his replacement at his place of work; and a new item of business for the undertaker; and so on and so on.) And similarly, an act of keeping a promise, or telling the truth, and so on, would be right or wrong not in itself, but in virtue of its consequences. But a different kind of theory denies what the consequentialist asserts. A ***deontological*** theory, as it is called, denies that the morality of an action is *solely* a matter of its consequences. This kind of theory can agree that the consequences of an action can matter morally, but it will insist that consequences are not the only things that matter. Rather, there are some actions that are right or wrong, as the case may be, just because of the kind of actions they are; they are right or wrong in themselves, or *intrinsically*. So, for instance, the act of killing an innocent person may be wrong just because it is the killing of an innocent person, regardless of its consequences. And an act of promise-keeping may be obligatory just because it is a case of promise-keeping, regardless of its consequences; and so on. According to the deontologist, we can have inescapable moral duties – to act as we are obliged to act, and to refrain from acting in ways that would be wrong – regardless of the consequences.

The consequentialist is surely correct to stress the moral significance of the consequences of our actions. We are often in some situation in which it is right to deliberate about the outcomes of the alternative courses of action open to us. How good would the outcome of this action be, and how good would be the alternative possible outcomes? What good and what bad can we identify in these alternative sets of consequences, and which set would be best overall? These can be very important moral questions, and it is surely true that our morally correct decision is often to be determined precisely by the answers to these questions. But is the deontologist correct to insist that consequences cannot be the *only* morally relevant consideration? The dispute here between consequentialist and deontologist is important, and we can get a grip on it by spending some time in considering the most prominent version of consequentialism – the theory called ***utilitarianism***.

Utilitarianism

Utilitarianism is enormously influential in philosophical ethics, particularly in philosophical contributions to applied and professional ethics. According to the basic kind of utilitarianism, there is one simple moral rule that we must obey at all times: each time that we make a decision how to act, we must choose, among the various possible actions that we could perform, that action whose consequences would involve *the greatest amount of good*. We must *maximise the good*. And this means bringing about the greatest *overall* amount of good. In the set of consequences of an action, there may be some good and some bad; and the overall amount of good is the net total there would be once the bad has been subtracted from the good. But now, what *is* the good that we must maximise? The answer given by classical utilitarianism is that the good is happiness, and the bad is suffering. So our moral duty is to bring about the greatest amount of happiness (as an overall, or net, amount – when the suffering is subtracted).

Let's see how this works in an imaginary case. Suppose that a friend of yours has borrowed some money from you, promising to pay it back at a certain time. And now that time has arrived. What ought your friend to do now? The deontologist may well say that (unless the circumstances are highly exceptional) the answer to this question is very straightforward: your friend ought to pay the money back to you, because it belongs to you and he promised to repay it now (for it's wrong not to keep our promises, and it's wrong to steal). But the utilitarian will say that the question cannot be answered so simply. According to the utilitarian, the answer will depend on how much good and bad there would be in the consequences of paying the money back to you now, on the one hand, and not paying it back to you now, on the other. So (according to the utilitarian) your friend needs to look ahead and predict the consequences of repaying it, and assess how much happiness there would be in those consequences, and subtract from that the amount of any suffering there would be in those consequences, and thus calculate the resultant net total of happiness (the happiness minus the suffering) that those consequences would contain. And he similarly needs to look ahead and calculate what net total of happiness there would be if he did *not* pay the money back. And then he needs to *compare* those different amounts, to see which course of action – paying it back or not paying it back – would lead to the *greatest* net total of happiness. And *that* will be the course of action he ought to pursue.

Of course, this calculation might take some doing. There would be some predictable good in the consequences of paying the money back to you. You would no doubt be caused some happiness in having the money returned to you and being able once again to use it as you decide. And there would be predictable bad in the consequences of not paying the money back. You would be caused some suffering, by being deprived of the money, and perhaps because of some breach of the friendship. And it may be that these goods and bads are such that the greatest good that your friend can do is to repay you the money now; and in that case the utilitarian decision about what to do will be the same as the deontologist's decision. But it will all depend on what the consequences would actually be. Perhaps your friend would also gain a lot of happiness by *keeping* the money, and wouldn't suffer much from a breach of the friendship. Or perhaps he could do a lot of good by giving the money, not to you, but to others; perhaps there is a good deal of happiness that he could cause if he gave the money to people who are in real need, and perhaps this happiness would certainly outweigh your happiness in using the money yourself, and would certainly offset your suffering in being deprived of it… According to the utilitarian, your friend needs to take all of this into account. He needs to do his best to assess the various possible outcomes, and then he needs to act to bring about the outcome which his assessment has indicated would involve the greatest amount of good. And thus his decision may or may not coincide with the deontologist's prescription about how to act.

Utilitarianism, as I have mentioned, is very influential in philosophical circles; and it is easy to see why some people find it powerfully attractive. It is a beautifully *simple* theory. It requires us to know, and follow, *merely one* simple moral rule: maximise the good. And, in appealing to that rule, it offers a simple *explanation* of what it is that makes something right or wrong. We ordinarily think that keeping promises and telling the truth and giving aid to someone in need, and so on, are right things to do; but utilitarianism can explain *why* they are right, *what it is* about these things that makes them the right thing to do – on those occasions, that is to say, when they *are* the right thing to do. And the theory brings morality down to earth, as it were. For it allows us to work out how to act merely by considering things that can be observed in the ordinary, natural world. In that respect, it is like egoism. But unlike egoism, it includes natural facts about others among the matters that I ought to be fundamentally concerned about. The first great utilitarian theorist, the 18th Century English philosopher Jeremy Bentham, said that the good is pleasure, and the bad is pain. Later utilitarians argued that this was too restrictive a notion of the good; and the most prominent of them, the 19th Century English philosopher John Stuart Mill, proposed that it should be replaced by the richer notion of happiness. And his version of utilitarianism – with happiness as the good and suffering as the bad – became the classical version. More recently, some utilitarians have argued that we need a yet richer notion of the good, to include the wide variety of things that people value or aim for in life – the things that people prefer. These utilitarians have proposed that the good comes about when people's preferences are satisfied, and so to maximise the good is to bring about the greatest overall total of satisfied preferences. But whichever of these notions of the good we work with – pleasure, happiness, the satisfaction of preferences – we are considering something that can actually be observed in people's lives in the natural world (and also in the lives of other sentient creatures – creatures that can *feel*). So we have a single simple rule, in application to ordinary observable goings-on; and in order to work out our moral duty, all we need to do is count up and weigh and compare these predictable natural possibilities. And I suspect that this way of thinking about morality is particularly attractive to those who might otherwise be worried by the thought that morality has some mysterious, perhaps even spooky, transcendental character; and especially by the thought that morality has some connection with religion.

We may or may not feel the attraction of those features. But in my own view, the most *nobly* attractive feature of utilitarianism is that it insists that we must consider the interests of *all* those who are affected by our actions. I am not permitted to do simply what suits me. When assessing the consequences of my possible courses of action, I must take into account the consequences for anyone and everyone who can be affected, and I must give full weight to their interests as well as to my own.

But whatever its attractions, utilitarianism is faced with formidable problems. First, though it is *theoretically* simple, it can *in practice* be nightmarishly complex and difficult. This may well have occurred to you as we considered the case of your friend working out whether to repay the loan. He needs, for a start, to *predict* the consequences of his various possible courses of action – *all* those consequences, however far they extend into the future. Then he needs to *identify* within those consequences the incidence of any possibly affected person's happiness (or preference-satisfaction, or whatever) or suffering. And then he needs to *measure* the *amounts* of those instances of happiness and suffering, and to *weigh* the different possible amounts against one another. And how is he to do all of this? Can he *really* predict all the consequences of his possible courses of action? And can he really tell where all the consequent happiness and suffering would lie? And how is he to measure those instances of happiness and suffering, and how is he to compare them? (How much happiness would there be – now, and into the indefinite future – if you and your family used the money to pay off some of your bank home loan? How much happiness would there be if your friend used the money to pay for his daughter's music lessons? How much happiness would there be if your friend spent the money on a series of gourmet meals accompanied by fine wines? How much happiness would there be if the money was sent as a contribution towards the digging of a well in a remote village in Africa? How much suffering would arise from a breach of your friendship? And so on, and so on. And can these amounts of happiness and suffering even *be* compared? Can we really weigh them against one another?) Still, the utilitarian might reply that these predictions and calculations are complicated just because real life is complicated. Morality is difficult because life is difficult. And any moral theory which suggests that the practice of morality is simple is a theory which fails to square up to the truth about life. So these difficulties for utilitarianism tend rather to indicate that it is the correct moral theory than otherwise. Well, is that a satisfactory reply? Do these problems tell for or against utilitarianism?

Another problem for the theory is connected with what I suggested was utilitarianism's noblest feature. The theory tells us that we must consider everyone who can be affected by our actions, and that my interests are no more important than anyone else's. It requires me to act in *whatever* way would produce the greatest amount of the good. And if I can do that by, for instance, giving my money to poor people whom I don't know on the other side of the world, then this is what I ought to do. Indeed, it seems that I ought to do so even to the extent that I end up no better off than they are (for while I remain wealthier than they are, there is yet more good that I can do with my money). So utilitarianism is very demanding – very uncomfortably demanding, because it will require many of us to make very great sacrifices. Still, the utilitarian can reply that morality *does* demand great sacrifice from those of us who are well off, so this is a point in the theory's favour, not against it. However, the problem gets worse. The theory demands that I sacrifice not only my own interests, but *also* the interests of the members of my family and others to whom I am particularly close. My daughter's interests, according to the utilitarian, are no more important than those of the unknown person on the other side of the world, so I have no greater duty towards her than to that unknown person. And the same is true of my wife's interests, or my son's, or my close friend's. If the greatest amount of good I can bring about involves giving to the unknown poor the money that I would otherwise have spent in looking after my family, then this is what I ought to do. But as many philosophers point out, this seems an unacceptable implication of utilitarianism, for the theory is here requiring us to abandon our *moral duties* towards those close to us. Again, the utilitarian can reply that here too, we have to grow up and take seriously the breadth of our moral obligations: we have to be prepared to make sacrifices not only of our own interests, but also of our selfish concerns for those near to us. But again, it is not at all clear that this is a satisfactory reply. We may well recognise that we have duties towards *anyone* in need, while also recognising that we have *special* duties towards those close to us (our family and friends, but also perhaps our employees, our patients, our clients, our students, and so on). And we may well feel that a man who considers that he has no special duties to his family is not someone who is to be congratulated for being unselfish; rather, he should be regarded as suffering some deep moral defect.

But in my view, the most serious problems facing utilitarianism can be seen by considering two well-known kinds of objection to the theory.

Here is an objection of the *first* kind. Imagine that in a certain country, there live many Nazis and fewer Jews. (And let's imagine that no-one else is affected by what happens in that country.) Now the Nazis would enjoy exquisite pleasure if they tortured and killed the Jews. (Or if you prefer, the Nazis would enjoy great happiness, or would have their preferences wonderfully satisfied, if they did that.) And the Nazis suffer considerable frustration while the Jews remain alive and well. The Jews, understandably enough, would enjoy their greatest pleasure (happiness, satisfaction of preferences) if they were allowed to get on with their lives undisturbed, and they would suffer very greatly if they were tortured and killed. But let's suppose that the *numbers* are such that the *greatest* net total of pleasure (happiness, etc.) would be brought about by the Nazis indeed torturing and killing the Jews. (That total will simply depend on the numbers – on there being a large enough number of Nazis, and few enough Jews, and the quantities of happiness and suffering that would be caused.) And in that case, the utilitarian will tell us – applying the rule that we must maximise the good – that the Nazis *ought* to torture and kill the Jews (and indeed that the Jews ought to allow themselves to be tortured and killed). But this would surely be morally wrong – indeed, outrageously wrong. And therefore utilitarianism is prescribing what is morally wrong; and therefore it is not a correct moral theory.

Let's note how this objection works by employing some of the tools of critical reasoning we gathered in Chapter Two. I have offered a *thought experiment*, by imagining a situation which allows us to put utilitarianism to the test. And the test gives us a result which we can present as a simple *argument*:

> *If utilitarianism is correct, then the Nazis (in the imagined case) ought to torture and kill the Jews.*
>
> *It is not the case that the Nazis (in the imagined case) ought to torture and kill the Jews.*
>
> ---
>
> *It is not the case that utilitarianism is correct.*

The argument has the clear conclusion that utilitarianism is incorrect. The argument is valid: it is, as you will recognise, an instance of modus tollens. And its premises seem to be true. The first premise simply applies the utilitarian rule to the situation described as imagined. And anyone who wishes to dispute the second premise will need to work very hard indeed to persuade the rest of us – to put it mildly. So the argument seems sound. And so it seems that we must accept the conclusion. And so it seems that the argument provides us with a falsification of utilitarianism.[4]

What might the utilitarian say in response? He (for convenience, I will refer to him as "he") might be tempted to protest that the real world is not like that imagined situation. In the real world, with its real numbers of people and the real things that make them happy or cause them to suffer, the numbers will not turn out as they are supposed to turn out in my imagined situation; and so in the real world, utilitarianism will not prescribe that appalling course of action. Well, he is of course correct to say that, fortunately enough, the real world is not like that – at least in many places (thanks to the efforts of our forebears), and for the time being. Nevertheless, his protest misses the point. For the success of the objection does not depend upon its pointing to an actual situation in the real world. The thought experiment can work because it points to a *possible* situation. Utilitarianism is proposed as a *general* moral theory, which is to say that it is supposed to deal with all possible moral situations. And so, if it prescribes what is wrong for a possible situation, it fails as a general moral theory.

Furthermore, the protest we have heard – that the numbers in the real world will fortunately turn out differently – fails to take seriously what the thought experiment shows about where utilitarianism goes wrong. For the problem is not merely that there are so many Nazis in that imagined situation, and that therefore we hear from the utilitarian rule an unpalatable prescription concerning what ought to be done. The problem, surely, is that utilitarianism is counting towards the good some things that ought not to be counted at all. The Nazi pleasure in torturing and killing Jews is not part of what ought to be counted as good! It is a *wicked* kind of pleasure, an *evil* pleasure. And any theory which proposes that taking pleasure in doing evil is the kind of thing that we ought to promote is surely a theory which has gone very badly wrong. (We might prefer to say that it is not the Nazis' pleasure *as such* that is not good, but the fact that the pleasure is enjoyed *in the doing of evil*. We can say this if we wish; but then it will remain true that pleasure taken in that sort of way is not part of the good that we ought to pursue, and the thought experiment remains fatal to utilitarianism because the theory regards *all* pleasure (happiness, etc.) as good. But in any case, the Nazis' pleasure is inseparable from what they do: it is inseparable from their torturing and killing of the

Jews. It is very artificial to try to imagine their pleasure except as part of the evil in which they engage.)

And note what this shows. We pointed out earlier that many people find utilitarianism attractive not least because it offers us a nicely down-to-earth account of what the good is – pleasure, or happiness, or preference-satisfaction – on the basis of which we can then work out how to assess the morality of all actions. But not all pleasure (or happiness etc.) deserves to be counted as good. Indeed, we can evaluate some kinds of pleasure (etc.) as morally *bad*. And the fact that we can evaluate different kinds of pleasure (etc.) in moral terms shows that we have a sense of what the good is that is quite independent of pleasure (etc.). If the good *just is* pleasure, then any pleasure counts as good; there can be no question of good or bad pleasures. But we can readily identify pleasures that we ought not to promote; so the good is not simply pleasure; so utilitarianism has not identified for us the basis of morality in the way it attempts to do. And its own basis collapses. And so we cannot rely on utilitarianism – at least in the form that we have so far considered – as an adequate moral guide.

I said that the most serious problems facing utilitarianism are displayed by two kinds of objection to the theory. We have just seen an instance of the first kind of objection. Now here is an objection of the *second* kind. Imagine that you are in charge of a surgical ward in a hospital. You have in your ward five patients who are desperately in need of organ transplants: two need a kidney transplant, one a heart, one a lung and one a liver; and all will die soon without the transplants. But there are no donor organs available. However, it so happens that there is a fit young woman walking outside, whose own organs would be compatible with your patients in need. You and your staff could ambush her, take her into the operating theatre, and redistribute her organs. It is true that you would thereby end her life. But you would save five lives for the cost of that one, and this is a terrific return on your investment. Here it seems obvious that the way to maximise the good is to seize that young woman and redistribute her organs, and so this is what utilitarianism would prescribe. But *would* that be right? Many of us would feel very deep qualms, to say the least. It is one thing, we might say, for someone to be prepared to donate an organ – even, perhaps, at the cost of her own life. But to seize a person, against her will, and kill her, and carve her up to redistribute her organs…! Wouldn't that be a particularly dreadful kind of murder? And wouldn't it be clearly wrong? And don't we, therefore, have another falsification of utilitarianism?

Once again, I have offered a thought experiment. And once again, it allows us to present a simple argument:

> *If utilitarianism is correct then it would be right (in the imagined case) to seize that young woman and kill her and redistribute her organs.*

It is not the case that it would be right (in the imagined case) to seize that young woman and kill her and redistribute her organs.

It is not the case that utilitarianism is correct.

And once again, the argument is valid. (It is an instance of modus tollens.) But is it sound? Does it provide a genuine falsification of utilitarianism?

If the utilitarian is to reject the argument, he must reject one of its premises. He might start by trying to reject the second premise. In other words, he might conclude that it would indeed be right to sacrifice the young woman. In concluding this, he would be biting the bullet, as we say, and accepting the surprising – indeed, shocking – implications of his theory. But if he does take this line, he will certainly need to work very hard indeed to persuade us that this is right. Many of us will feel that he has here a hopeless task.

But he might reject the first premise. He might say that utilitarianism does *not* require us to sacrifice that young woman. How might he say this? Well, he could direct our attention to consequences that I have not considered thus far. He might point out that we need to consider not only the young woman's own suffering and the loss of the good that she would herself have enjoyed in her future life, but also the suffering that her death would cause to her family and friends, and the loss of the good that she would have done for others in the future, and the alarm and distress caused to the hospital staff by the procedures required for her sacrifice, and so on. And we have to keep in mind that it is unlikely that one person could provide all the compatible organs required for five different patients; so finding the required organs would probably require the sacrifice of more lives than I have imagined. And the utilitarian might say that when we do consider all these further consequences, and make a more accurate calculation, it is not clear that the young woman's sacrifice would maximise the good after all, and so it is not clear that utilitarianism does have that shocking implication.

Now of course, the utilitarian is quite right to insist that *all* consequences be taken into account. That is what his theory requires. And it is no doubt true that in many situations of the kind being imagined, the young woman's sacrifice would indeed have such further unfortunate consequences. But we can tweak the thought experiment in such a way that those bad consequences are minimised. (We need only to imagine a *possible* situation, after all.) So let us suppose that this young woman has no family and few friends, and that she is, I'm afraid, the sort of person who is unlikely to make any great contribution to the future happiness of others; though she is, fortunately, able to supply all the required organs. And let us suppose that the required team of hospital staff are well trained in acting, without qualms or undue sensitivity, for the greatest good, and so are committed to performing the ambush and surgical procedures efficiently and *quietly*, without drawing any attention to what they are doing, and thus causing minimal pain to the young woman (who is speedily anaesthetised) and minimal alarm or distress to anyone else… And so on. In other words, we can imagine circumstances in which the young woman's sacrifice really does maximise the good, and so that it really is what utilitarianism prescribes.

Even so, the utilitarian can still insist that we haven't yet considered all the consequences. He might, more or less begrudgingly, accept that there could be *the odd occasion* on which a sacrifice like this could maximise the good in its particular set of circumstances. But, he can say, this can't often be the case. And he has powerful reasons for saying this. For let us think seriously about what would happen once it is known that the hospital team does practise this kind of sacrifice. Though the team may wish to perform the procedures quietly, they would inevitably become known throughout the hospital, as staff talk; and among the wider public, as family and friends of those who are sacrificed made increasingly noisy enquiries concerning the disappearance of their loved ones. The public would surely be deeply alarmed. And the real cause for concern here is not just that the public would protest at the hospital practice; for we can perhaps imagine that the hospital, and the relevant public lawmakers, could come to *accept* this practice for hard-headed utilitarian reasons, and seek to persuade the public also to accept it, on the ground that this is the way we must all be prepared to work for the greatest good. The real cause for concern, the utilitarian can say, is that the hospital system would cease to function properly; it would cease to fulfil its *general* purpose to heal the sick and thereby work towards the greatest good. For ask yourself what you would do if you broke your wrist, but knew that if you presented yourself at the local emergency department, there would be a fair chance that you would never emerge because you would be spirited off to theatre to have all your organs redistributed. And ask yourself whether you would present yourself with the symptoms of a highly infectious disease. (The hospital could put you in quarantine, give you the treatment to cure you, and *then* spirit you off to theatre…) Ask yourself, indeed, whether you would ever wish to go anywhere near a hospital at all, whether you were sick or well. The real concern, the utilitarian can insist, is that public knowledge of the hospital's preparedness to redistribute organs would cause people to lose all trust in hospitals for their own care, and this would have the consequence that those who were sick would not be treated, and so they would suffer and many would die; and these sick people would also cause wider suffering to others, through infection, and because of the burden they would impose upon ordinary members of the public. The policy of non-voluntary redistribution of organs would therefore cause great harm, the utilitarian can say, and so it is not required by his theory. And therefore that argument seeking to falsify the theory is in fact unsound: its first premise is not true.

These are very important considerations. And it is through reasoning just like this that some utilitarians *modify* their theory in a way we should note. These utilitarians stress that, for just these reasons, we need to consider the consequences of *policies and general practices*, not of particular actions. The basic kind of utilitarianism by which I have introduced the theory tells us that, for each action we perform, we must consider whether *that particular action* maximises the good. But the modified version of utilitarianism tells us to ask what *kind* of action would maximise the good if we performed it *over the long run*. Consider again the case we have just been thinking about. If we were looking only at the particular action of redistributing that young woman's organs, as an isolated event, we might conclude that it would maximise the good. But if we ask about the consequences of performing that kind of action *repeatedly*, within its wider context, we realise that, for the reasons we have just seen, this would cause great harm. In order to maximise the good *in the long term*, we need instead to observe *a policy, or a general rule*, which says something like "Don't perform non-voluntary redistribution of organs". So this modified version of utilitarianism holds that, although there is only one *fundamental* moral rule – namely, maximise the good – there are various *other* rules that we must obey. For, by repeatedly obeying these other (secondary) rules, we will, over the long term, maximise the good; and thereby, in the great scheme of things, obey the fundamental moral rule. This modified version of the theory, because it holds that we must obey a whole range of moral rules (which is how we maximise the good), is called ***rule utilitarianism***. The basic version of the theory, on the other hand, tells us that we can ignore any rule other than the one utilitarian rule (to maximise the good), and that we must apply this rule to every action that we perform. This basic kind of utilitarianism is called ***act utilitarianism***.

Many of us are far more comfortable with rule utilitarianism than with act utilitarianism. For rule utilitarianism turns out to prescribe much of what we ordinarily think that morality prescribes. (We have seen how it can tell us not to perform non-voluntary redistribution of organs. But we can imagine it making a similar case for such rules as "Don't kill innocent persons", "Don't steal", "Tell the truth", "Keep your promises", "Look after your family", and so on.) And we may be attracted by its utilitarian claim that it can show us *why* those rules are the right rules to follow. It claims that the reason for keeping these rules is that by doing so, we advance the greatest good, and so it persists in utilitarianism's promise to take the mystery out of morality.

Nevertheless, in my view, rule utilitarianism is not a satisfactory moral theory; and to show why it is not, I wish to extend my thought experiment a little further. Let's imagine that the hospital team, aware of the need to preserve the public's trust, certainly does not pursue an open policy of non-voluntary redistribution of organs, and indeed denies that anything so dreadful as such a policy is even contemplated. However, the team are very well trained, and committed to doing the greatest good; and they are actually committed, despite their denials, to being ready to perform organ redistributions, *but only* on those occasions when there is such a need *and* when the team really can preserve the *secrecy* of their procedures. They find the required organs by seizing fit but homeless people, who will not be missed by others; and their procedures, when performed, are skilfully concealed from other members of staff and from the wider public. (The organ recipients are told that they receive donor organs in the usual way.) And now let us suppose that these are the circumstances when our earlier situation arises. Five lives can be saved for the cost of that young woman's life. And there will be no public alarm, or other unfortunate consequences, for no-one will miss the young woman, and the whole procedure will be performed under a thoroughly effective veil of secrecy. And now I pose *a question for the rule utilitarian.* What should be done in this case?

The rule utilitarian here has a choice. He can say either that the young woman should be killed and her organs redistributed, or that she should not be interfered with (and the five patients die). Which does he choose? He would normally say, for the reasons we heard, that we should follow the rule that tells us *not* to seize anyone for organ redistribution. But should he say that *now*? He might well point out that now, in the situation as described, there is no longer any *utilitarian reason* to follow that rule. Following that rule in *this* situation would simply get in the way of achieving the greatest good. The way to maximise the good here is to sacrifice the young woman and save the five lives. And this, I think, *if he is being true to his utilitarianism*, is what he will say. And so here, as a genuine utilitarian, he will prescribe that we ignore that usual rule and simply perform the action that will maximise the good – by sacrificing the young woman. Here, in other words, the *rule* part of rule utilitarianism falls away, and it reverts to act utilitarianism.

But he could choose the other answer. He might say that in this situation, even though we have ensured that there would be no overriding harmful consequences of the sacrifice of the young woman, we should still stick to the rule *not* to engage in non-voluntary organ redistribution. He might say that the rule still applies. And if he does say this, he will be saying what many of us certainly feel. We feel that it would be very wrong – outrageously wrong – to seize that young woman and kill her for that purpose (much as we wish we could save those five patients). So if the rule utilitarian does here stick to the rule, then his view lines up with what ordinary morality will say. However, if he does say this, then *he has given up any utilitarian reason for his prescription*. The whole point of the situation, as I have now described it, is that now it gives us no utilitarian reason for obeying that rule there. And so, if the rule utilitarian still feels that the right thing to do is to keep obeying that rule, then I think he shows that he is not really a utilitarian at all.

Let's note how my argument here works. I have presented the rule utilitarian with a *dilemma*. He can choose one or the other of two options, but either choice is costly for him. His first option is to recognise that in the situation as described, there is no utilitarian reason for obeying the rule against organ redistribution; and hence, sticking to his guns as a utilitarian, he can ignore the rule and prescribe that the young woman be sacrificed. This option is consistent with his utilitarianism. But it is inconsistent with what we typically believe to be right. For most of us, I think, believe that the sacrifice would be wrong – very wrong indeed. So the cost of this option, for the utilitarian, is that his theory has a consequence that we find unacceptable. His other option is to say that it would indeed be wrong to sacrifice the young woman, for we should follow the normal rule, or rules, against such a course of action. This option makes what he says consistent with ordinary morality. But it seems to me to be inconsistent with utilitarianism, for, in the situation as now described, there is no utilitarian reason for this option, and indeed the fundamental utilitarian rule would tell us *not* to choose this option. So it seems to me that the cost of this option, for the utilitarian, is that he gives up his utilitarianism. In taking this option, his view merges with the more ordinary morality maintained by the rest of us. (And in taking this option, he shows himself, it seems to me, to be better than his theory.)

So, one way or the other, rule utilitarianism falls away. Either it merges into a more ordinary non-utilitarian moral outlook or it reverts back to act utilitarianism. And thus, it seems to me, rule utilitarianism disappears from the theoretical field we need to be examining.

We are left, then, with act utilitarianism as the live theoretical option within the utilitarian camp. And we have already seen the problems it faces. Let us remind ourselves of those problems. The theory will be fiendishly difficult to apply in practice. It faces real trouble in trying to account for our special moral duties towards those closest to us. And it appears to be confronted by fatal objections from the two arguments I presented, for in the situations imagined, it prescribes actions – the Nazi torture and killing of the Jews, and the killing of the young woman for the redistribution of her organs – which would surely be very wrong. As we think about those objections, what can we say about *why* the prescribed actions are wrong? *How is it* that they are wrong? We see that the utilitarian is working with an inadequate idea of what the good is, for such happiness as is enjoyed by the Nazis in their wicked activities ought not to count as good; it ought not to count as the sort of thing we should promote. And the wrongness of the prescribed actions – the torture and killing of the Jews, the sacrifice of the young woman – can be described in a variety of ways. We might say that these actions would breach certain moral *rules*, or *principles* – such as that it is wrong to inflict unnecessary pain, that it is wrong to kill innocent persons, and so on. We might say that these actions violate certain *rights* – the Jews' and the young woman's right not to be interfered with, their right to life, and so on. We might say that these actions would involve a gross lack of respect for the Jews' and young woman's *human dignity*... And we might think about whether one of those ways of stating what we believe is better than the other ways. But all of those things can be said; and in saying any of them, we are agreeing with what the *deontologist* says against the utilitarian in particular. For whichever way we put it, we are saying that those actions would be wrong regardless of their consequences. We are saying that those actions would be *intrinsically* wrong, wrong in themselves. And this shows that we accept that utilitarianism cannot be a fully satisfactory theory of morality, for it stands in need of correction from a deontological moral outlook.

In this discussion of the pros and cons of the theory of utilitarianism, we have been deploying some of the critical equipment gathered in Chapter Two. We have been *testing the theory by examining some of its consequences*. We have designed some *thought experiments* which allow us to assess the consequences of utilitarianism over and against the consequences of a deontological account of morality; and we have discovered places where, it seems to me, we need to reject the consequences of utilitarianism, and, in rejecting those consequences, to evaluate them in just the way that a deontological account of morality does evaluate them. These points can be expressed as *arguments* that can be set out so that they can be tested for *validity*, and their premises for *truth*. And in all of this, we have been engaging in an exercise of *reflective equilibrium*. We have been balancing what the theories say against what our own moral sense, our own moral intuitions, tell us. I have been arguing that our own moral sense shows that some of what utilitarian theory prescribes is wrong, and therefore that we should reject the theory. The hard-headed utilitarian might perhaps reply, by contrast, that his theory does indeed have consequences that clash with our ordinary moral sense, and therefore that we should reject our ordinary moral sense. (He might claim that it is right for those Nazis to torture and kill the Jews, and for the hospital team to sacrifice that young woman.) He might claim that our ordinary moral intuitions need to be revised under the guidance of his theory. (You can set out his reasoning in arguments which have the form of modus ponens.) Whereas I claim that his theory needs to be revised under the guidance of our ordinary moral intuitions. (My reasoning can be expressed, as we have seen, as arguments which have the form of modus tollens. And, because I take these arguments to be sound, I take his arguments to be unsound. In particular, the second premise in his arguments, which asserts that utilitarianism is correct, is shown by my arguments to be false.) And I hope that my view is shared by others.

And so I conclude that utilitarianism is an unsatisfactory moral theory. It needs, at least, to be supplemented, or balanced, by deontological considerations. And this means that we cannot expect utilitarianism to provide an adequate framework for the ethics of the caring professions.

Distinctive features of professional ethics, and a particular clash with utilitarianism

However, it seems to me that there is still a further, *particular* reason why utilitarianism does not provide the right way to think about the ethics of professional care. It is an important reason, which emerges from what we have already noted about utilitarianism. But to see it clearly, we need to take a short detour to the side and think about what a profession is and why it requires its own code of ethics.

What is a profession? The title "profession" is nowadays attached to an increasingly long list of activities. But it was traditionally given to a few select occupations, which shared a number of particular characteristics; and it seems to me sensible to continue to use the term in more or less that narrower sense, because by doing so, we can identify something of special importance. The traditional professions (medicine, law, ordained ministry within the Christian church, and later other occupations too) were regarded as special in the following ways. First, each of them was devoted to an activity intended to provide a service of great importance in human life and society – the saving of life; the preserving of health; the ordering of personal life and of our relations with one another in ways that are regarded as deeply significant. Secondly, they all required their members to undergo lengthy and rigorous study and training in order to acquire an adequate level of competence in their field, because the performance of the service to which the occupation was devoted depended upon its members possessing that level of quite particular and special competence. Thirdly, the professions required their members to subscribe to particular standards of conduct in the performance of their occupation. Often this requirement involved commitment to a formal code of professional ethics – sometimes in the form of an oath, or a vow. And fourthly, the professions regulated themselves, at least to a considerable extent. Among other things, they themselves determined the standard of learning and the standard of conduct required for membership of their profession.

Now why is it that the professions have had this particular commitment to their own ethics, and to their self-regulation? To see this, let us think for a moment not about the relation between a professional and his or her client, but about an ordinary transaction in the traditional marketplace. Imagine that you are looking to buy a piece of cloth, or a horse. There is a vendor who wishes to sell; you wish to buy. And each of you wishes to be sure that you will get what you want from the transaction: you wish to ensure that the cloth, or the horse, is of the quality you require; while the vendor wishes to ensure that you will be good for the purchase price. And each of you can take steps to assure yourselves. The vendor can ask to see the colour of your money. You can measure and examine the cloth, or look the horse in the mouth. Thus, each of you is in a position to take effective practical steps to protect your own interests. Still, there is some risk. For instance, the horse's condition may not be as sound as it seems. The vendor's thumb may be covering a hole in the cloth. And so we need to keep in mind the old maxim *caveat emptor* – "let the buyer beware". Of course, modern society has progressively added various legal protections for both vendor and purchaser, and we have invented instruments such as warranties, and so on. But the basic idea of a transaction in the marketplace still assumes that buyer and seller stand on a roughly equal footing, for each is in a position to protect his own interests.

But now compare the relation, say, between a surgeon and her patient. You are dependent on your surgeon for something of enormous importance – the preservation of your life (not for a piece of cloth or a horse which can be bought and sold). And you are not in a position to protect your own interests as the transaction unfolds. Of course, you might ask around beforehand, seeking from your acquaintances their recommendation of a good surgeon. But as you go under the anaesthetic, you will certainly be in no position to check the quality of your surgeon's performance (even if you possessed the relevant knowledge, which you would not possess unless you had attained surgical expertise yourself). So what guarantee is there that your interests *will* be protected? Only the surgeon herself can provide that guarantee. Only she can ensure that she is performing the operation with the required expert skill, and only she can ensure that she is performing it in a way that is aimed at your best interests. And it makes sense for you to undergo the operation only if you can *trust her* to conduct herself in just that way. What is true of your surgeon is true also of other professionals – other doctors, lawyers, and so on. Only they can ensure that what they are doing is providing the service you need in the way you need. You have to trust them to conduct themselves with adequate expertise and in protection of your best interests. (Of course, it might *later* be discovered that they have failed to do this. But then it may be too late for you, or anyone, to rectify the situation. It may be too late for you to be healed of the side-effects of the wrongly prescribed medicine. It may be too late for the money lost from the trust fund to be recovered, or for you to get back the years of life spent in prison because of negligent defence at your trial. And it will certainly be too late for you to prevent the botched operation which caused you to die on the operating table, or for you to rewrite your will so that it turns out to accomplish what you had thought it would accomplish.)

The professions, of course, understand this. They know that the proper performance of the service they offer depends on each professional's competence and conduct. It is up to the professional to ensure that your interests are protected. And it is up to the profession to ensure that its members can perform with adequate competence and with the necessary commitment to the good of those they serve. For no one else has the required expertise for this to be assessed. There are many situations where members of the profession themselves are the only kind of people who can tell whether someone can perform, and is performing, in the way the profession expects.

And that is why the professions need to regulate themselves. (At least to some extent. Their regulation can be reinforced by wider public law. But even so, the public authorities will need to rely on members of the profession to determine what counts as properly competent performance within the profession.) And as part of their self-regulation, the professions typically formulate their own professional code of ethics, which they require their members to observe. The members openly *commit themselves* to these ethical standards, so that the profession, and the wider public which it serves, can see that they have made these standards their own. For the profession understands that we members of the public will be able to trust their members for their service only if we are sure that they are committed to the expected standard of performance. Their commitment provides the basis of our trust. They have made this public promise to maintain those standards and protect our interests, and, relying on that promise, we commit ourselves and our interests to their care.

Professional ethical codes tend to vary between the different professions. But they overlap in the promises they make. They typically promise that the members of the profession will act in the patient's (or client's) best interests; that they will avoid doing anything that will jeopardise the patient's (or client's) welfare; that they will ensure that the patient (or client) is fully provided with relevant information and advice, and willingly consents to whatever is done; that confidentiality will be preserved; and so on. Of course, these promises may be subject to various qualifications, but those qualifications will themselves be governed by other ethical principles. So for instance, the professional will act in my best interest *so long as* by doing so he or she does not wrongly undermine the interests of others – for example, by violating the rights of some other person. And the professional will gain my informed consent *where* this is possible. (It would not be possible, for example, if I were unconscious, but in desperate need of some surgical intervention.) And the professional will preserve confidentiality *so long as* this would not endanger someone else. (It would be dangerous, for example, if I had revealed that I intended to murder someone.) The professions, and we members of the public, understand that the promises are subject to such ethical qualifications. And it is on these promises that we members of the public rely when we place our trust in the professional.

Now I said a little while ago that there is a particular reason why utilitarianism does not square with professional ethics. What is that reason? We have just observed that each profession requires its members to commit themselves to a certain standard of conduct, and that this is the basis for our trust in their care, and therefore for their delivery of their care. And the rule utilitarian will readily endorse what we have just been observing. He might say that we have been observing an example of the very thing he describes – namely, that each profession serves a great good, and its doing so depends upon its members all promising to follow various moral rules, or principles ("Act in the patient's best interest", "Act only with properly informed consent", "Preserve confidentiality", and so on). Now the rule utilitarian is quite correct to note *this*. But I have argued that his rule utilitarian theory collapses (for he has no *utilitarian* reason to follow those rules when he can maximise the good by flouting them). Genuine utilitarianism reverts to act utilitarianism. And the act utilitarian is a *calculator*. He is at each point calculating which course of action would bring about the best consequences. So, for example, he will make a promise only when he calculates that by doing so he will maximise the good. He might calculate that by making a particular promise and then keeping it, he will maximise the good. Or he might calculate that by making the promise, he can achieve the good in some *other* way. For instance, and to recall our extreme example, if by making a promise to act in my best interests he can entice me into the operating theatre, where he can then redistribute my organs, he might calculate that making that promise is his means to maximising the good. But if he does keep a promise, it will not be because he believes in the moral principle that we ought to keep our promises. He will make promises, and keep them or otherwise, only when he calculates that by doing so he will maximise the good. So he does not believe in making the kinds of promises entailed by the professional codes, for those codes require him to *bind himself* always to conduct himself in certain ways. Of course, he might calculate that he can maximise the good by *saying* that he so binds himself (without intending in fact to be bound); but in that case he is engaged in deception.

And nor does he believe in the particular provisions of the code. He does not believe that he should always act in the patient's best interests. He believes that he should act in that way only when the patient's best interests coincide with the greatest good. And when he is prepared to act in a way that is contrary to my interests, it is not because he believes that he needs to observe someone else's rights, for he does not believe in rights. (As we noted earlier, rights are a deontological idea, for the notion of a right entails that some actions would be intrinsically right or wrong.) Nor does he believe that he should always obtain my informed consent to what he intends to do. If he believes that he can maximise the good by lying to me, or by coercing me, then this is what he will believe that he should do. (To return to our extreme example, he might believe that he can maximise the good by redistributing my organs, and he can get me into theatre for that purpose by lying to me about the treatment I will receive, or by seizing me and forcing me there.) And whether he preserves my confidentiality, and so on, will depend, as ever, on the calculation he makes in the particular circumstances.

So the utilitarian does not believe in making promises in the way the professional codes require. And he does not believe in the particular principles enshrined in the codes. Indeed, some utilitarian philosophical colleagues of mine have told me that in their view, this whole traditional view of professional ethics ought to be abandoned.

But it gets worse. Let's imagine that a utilitarian way of thinking does become more prominent in discussion of professional ethics. And imagine how this alters the expectations of the members of the public. We come to understand that the professionals whose service we need do not believe in binding themselves to the conduct described in the traditional codes. Indeed, we come to understand that even if they apparently *promise* to conduct themselves in those ways, they may be merely *saying* that they are making that promise only because they calculate that by doing so they can pursue the greatest good (and the greatest good may be contrary to our individual interests, and it may be contrary to what we might regard as our own or any other individual's rights). In fact, we come to understand that *anything* the professionals say to us may *or may not* be true, for they will tell the truth only when they calculate that by doing so they can maximise the good. Under these circumstances, can we *trust* professionals in the way we need to do if we are to surrender to their care? It seems dreadfully clear that we cannot. But if we cannot trust them, we have no basis on which to submit to their care. But then their professional service collapses, and the great good to which the profession is devoted cannot be achieved.

At this point, the rule utilitarian might wish to pop up again and protest. Doesn't this show, he might repeat, that the way to *maximise the good* is, after all, for the professionals to *follow those rules* prescribed in their codes? But – once again – I have already argued that rule utilitarianism fails. And what we have just seen does not show that rule utilitarianism is correct; it does not answer my earlier argument. The rule utilitarian wants to explain what we have just been observing about the professions by saying that *what makes the professional rules morally correct* is that *by* following them we can attain the greatest good. But that is to put it the wrong way around. (If that were the right way to put it, then it would no longer be correct to follow the rules when we can achieve the greatest good by violating them; and so it would, for instance, be right to kill that young woman and redistribute her organs when we really can do so in complete secrecy.) The right way to put it is surely this: the professional moral rules are morally correct rules, and when they are faithfully followed, the profession can successfully provide the service to which it is devoted. The great good of professional care can be provided because the members of the profession observe rules that are correct in themselves – *intrinsically* correct. When the professionals bind themselves to these rules, we members of the public can trust them for our care; and when we trust them, they can deliver that care and thereby serve a great good. It is not that the correctness of the rules depends upon their leading to the great good. It is rather that the achievement of the great good depends upon the professionals reliably observing the correct rules. It depends upon the professionals conducting themselves, as we put it, with *integrity*.

And thus we see this further particular reason to regard utilitarianism as an unsatisfactory theory: it cannot provide the framework for professional ethics. The practice of utilitarianism would in fact undermine the possibility of professional service. We need to regard professional ethics in *deontological* terms – as the observance of various rules or principles that are correct in themselves. And successful professional service requires the professionals to *bind themselves* to these rules. We members of the public need to be able to regard the professional as someone whom we can *trust*; as someone *upon whom we can rely* in that way. We need *reliable* professionals – persons who do not merely parrot the rules, but have *made those rules their own*. Following those rules has become part of their *character*. So the professional needs to be *a certain kind of person*. And that brings us to one further philosophical theory which we need to note before concluding this chapter.

Virtues and character

Early in this chapter, I contrasted a consequentialist moral theory (of which the most prominent and influential example is utilitarianism) with a deontological moral theory. But there is also another kind of non-consequentialist moral theory. This theory holds that what makes an action right or wrong is not its set of consequences, but the character of the person who performs the action. The key idea in a theory of this kind is the idea of a ***virtue***. What is a virtue? It is *an admirable, or worthy, character trait*. So the virtues would include the following: courage, loyalty, honesty, benevolence (a concern and willingness to act for the good of others), generosity, justice, fairness, compassion, tact, considerateness, sensitivity, humility, self-control, patience, kindness, reliability, faithfulness, diligence, prudence, responsibility, self-reliance, strength, endurance… That list is in no particular order, and it is certainly not complete. Just as we have such terms for the virtues ("courage", "loyalty", etc.), we also have terms for failure of virtue ("cowardice", "disloyalty", "dishonesty", "thoughtlessness", "unkindness", "unfairness", "callousness", "cruelty", "meanness", "selfishness", "weakness", "intemperance", etc.). And where a failure of virtue is itself a trait of character, it has become a *vice*. But how can the idea of a virtue become the key idea in a whole theory of morality? Since the ancient Greeks, there have been philosophers who have maintained that what makes an action right or wrong is whether it is an action that the fully virtuous person would perform. For the virtues are character traits that we all ought to be developing in ourselves – traits that we develop by *practising* the kind of action they entail, and in that way forming such *habits* within ourselves. (How, for instance, do we become courageous? By practising courage; by practising acting well in response to danger and difficulty, and thereby developing the habit of acting in that way. Through such practice, we make it *more natural* for ourselves to act in that way.) The kind of person that we all *ought to be* is the person who possesses all the virtues; and so the kind of thing we all *ought to do* is what would be done by that fully virtuous person. Thus, when we need to know how we ought to act in some situation, we should ask: what would the fully virtuous person do in this situation? And so this kind of theory can give us a rule for all conduct. How ought we to act? *We should act in the way that the fully virtuous person would act.*

But can such a theory provide a fully satisfactory account of morality? In particular, can it tells us *why* we should be virtuous? Those who have favoured this kind of theory – particularly Aristotle, its greatest champion – have stressed that we need to possess the virtues if we are going to achieve what is worthwhile in life. If my character fails in respect of one or other of the virtues, I am likely to miss out on what matters. And it is easy to see examples of this, as we think about various virtues. Consider courage once again. I will need to possess courage not only if I am to get through situations of physical danger, but also if I am to deal well with many other kinds of unpleasant situation that need to be faced. Or consider loyalty. Without loyalty, I will be unable to enjoy to the full the family relationships and friendships that I would wish for. And so on. But can we build up a *complete* account of morality in this way? If we concentrate on trying to demonstrate that we need the virtues in order to attain what we *want* in life, then our account is in danger of degenerating into a story about our own self-interest; and such a story, as we saw when we were discussing egoism, is a morally defective story. But we can avoid egoism if we claim that the virtues are required for what is worthwhile in life, what matters, *and* we include in what matters what we *ought* to be seeking in life, including the good of others. (And we can add that the best life *for us* is the life that also involves a proper concern *for others*.) However, if we *do* include what we ought to be seeking and doing as part of our account of the worthwhile life, then we are *already* working with notions of what we *ought* to be doing – notions with which we are operating, but which make no reference to the virtues. So those notions of what we ought to do have to come from somewhere other than our story about the need for the virtues. And this, I think, is the case. Thus, for instance, if we ask why the virtue of benevolence is required, our answer will need to include the fact that we have duties to act for the good of others, even on occasions when that is to our own cost. And if we ask why the virtue of honesty is required, our answer will need to include the fact that we have duties of truthfulness to others, even on occasions when telling the truth will disadvantage us. And so on. Furthermore, if we are to spell out what a particular virtue requires, we may well need to refer to rules or principles that are properly understood in deontological terms. For instance, a person cannot act *justly* unless he can recognise the *rights* that are possessed by the different people in the relevant situation.

In other words, it seems to me that a stress upon the virtues needs to work along with, and be informed by, a wider recognition of our moral duties. In particular, it needs to recognise rules and principles that are best expressed in deontological terms. And if that is correct, then a theory of the virtues cannot provide a *complete* theory of morality, but it *overlaps* with insights from other theories.

And in my view, a stress on the virtues complements what other theories offer in two particularly helpful respects. First, it can help us to think about moral questions by employing a richer set of resources than we might otherwise use. As we noted in Chapter One, we need not ask simply whether some action would be right or wrong. We can ask morally relevant questions about our personal characteristics, including the traits of character from which an action might naturally spring. And in asking what the *fully* virtuous person would do, we remind ourselves that there may well be a *variety* of ways in which our acting needs to be right. It may need, for example, to be adequately *courageous*, but *also* adequately *compassionate*, *and* adequately *fair*. And similarly, there can be a variety of ways in which our acting can go wrong. It may be cowardly; or it may be cruel or mean or hard-hearted; or it may be unfair; or it may be some combination of these. And so on. We thus remind ourselves of the *range* of moral requirements, and we have a set of tools to help us to *pinpoint* just where we can go right or wrong – a set of tools that is much more informative than the bald words "right" and "wrong".

And the second helpful advantage of a stress upon the virtues arises from what we have already noted. Only if we embody *all* the virtues can we be *relied upon* to act as we ought to act in *whatever* situation that may arise. But we *embody* a virtue only when it is part of our character. The person who has *become* courageous is someone who can be relied upon to face danger or unpleasantness properly whenever it crops up, even if it has not been foreseen. The person who has become compassionate can be relied upon to respond with properly sympathetic care whenever someone in need appears, however unexpectedly. And so on. Now we saw how important it is that professionals be people who can be relied upon, *trusted*, to act in the various ways that their profession demands. And so we see that professional ethics requires not only that professionals *subscribe* to the relevant ethical principles, but that they have *made those principles their own by making them part of their character*. In other words, the principles which the professionals have promised to follow need to be transformed into *virtues* embodied by the professionals themselves. The professionals who embody these virtues display *professional integrity*: they display a wholeness and completeness; there is a sound and dependable consistency between what they say and what they do because of the kind of person they *are*. And in seeing this, we see, I think, a particularly important aspect of professional ethics.

Conclusion

It turns out, then, that a variety of philosophical theories make useful contributions to our understanding of professional ethics. We have just seen the importance of a concentration on the virtues. We have repeatedly seen that there are inescapable moral requirements which need to be understood deontologically. And though I have been very critical of utilitarianism, we can recognise that a serious concern for the consequences of our actions may indeed be morally required, so long as we do not regard it as the only morally relevant factor.

If utilitarianism were true, then moral requirements could be set out within a very simple system, for there would be only one moral rule that we would need to apply – the rule to maximise the good. (Though the practical application of this rule would in fact be frightfully complex.) But we have seen powerful reasons to reject utilitarianism; and in recognising those reasons, we have noted a *range* of rules or principles which state what is intrinsically right or wrong. These constitute the deontological core of morality. However, we have not yet managed to gather these rules into a collection which has any systematic shape. Nor have we done much to spell out their detailed application to the caring professions. The next chapter should help us to make some progress in both those directions.

Notes

1 Thomas Hobbes, *Leviathan*, Part 1, Chapter 13, paragraph 9.
2 *The Gospel according to Matthew*, 7:12, and elsewhere.
3 *The Gospel according to Mark*, 12:31, and elsewhere.
4 This modus tollens argument, as we learned in Chapter Two, seeks to refute utilitarianism by pointing to the fact that the theory has a false *consequence*. And utilitarianism is a theory which holds that only the *consequences* of actions are relevant to their morality. We may become uneasy about the different ways in which the word "consequence" is now being used. But we need not be troubled, for it is the right word in each case. In talking about the *consequences of an action*, the moral consequentialist is referring to the *actual effects* that would be brought about if the action occurred in the real world. But when we are considering the *consequences of a view or theory*, we are looking at what would be true if the view or theory were true, which includes logical consequences. Each kind of consequence can be reported by a conditional proposition. "If the Nazis torture and kill the Jews, then the Nazis will experience exquisite pleasure" is a conditional of the former kind – stating an effect of the action. "If utilitarianism is correct then the Nazis ought to torture and kill the Jews" is a conditional of the latter kind – stating a consequence of the theory. There will be times when we are discussing the consequences of actions. And there will be times when we are discussing the consequences of a theory or view, and in particular we will be using those consequences to help us test the theory. As long as we keep in mind what we are doing at each point, we need not become confused.

5
Four principles

In our discussion so far, we have recognised a number of different rules or principles which state moral requirements. But we have identified these rules in only a piecemeal fashion. And we have not yet managed to construct from them any kind of system, or framework, which allows us to see the rules in their correct relations to each other, and which can guide us in the detail of their application within the practical circumstances of the caring professions.

An ethical framework

In fact, such a framework has already been proposed and for some decades has been very commonly appealed to across the caring professions. It is a framework which consists of four ethical principles – the principles of beneficence, of non-maleficence, of respect for autonomy, and of justice. These four principles are particularly prominent in current ethical discussion because, according to many people, they usefully simplify the subject and help us to get some systematic grip on practical moral problems. What are these principles about, exactly?

"Beneficence" means "doing good", so the principle of beneficence is the principle that we ought to act for the good of others. "Maleficence" means "doing harm", so the principle of non-maleficence requires us to avoid doing harm to others. "Autonomy" means "self-rule", so the principle of respect for autonomy is the principle that we ought to respect and support others to determine for themselves what happens to them. And the principle of justice requires that we act justly.

The idea that we ought to act in these ways is as old as morality itself; but in the contemporary discussion, the four principles have been made famous by American ethicists Tom Beauchamp and James Childress. Their book *Principles of Biomedical Ethics* was first published in 1979. Its Eighth Edition was published in 2019.[1] It has become the most famous book in healthcare ethics and it has been hugely influential since it was first published. Beauchamp and Childress

DOI: 10.4324/9781003176541-6

use the four principles to provide what they believe is the right framework within which to understand and tackle biomedical ethical problems. But the influence of their book has gradually extended beyond the bounds of healthcare, for the framework they provide has also been found useful by members of other caring professions, including social work, social welfare and so on.

Not everyone believes that the four-principles framework provides the best way to think about professional ethics in the caring professions. Beauchamp and Childress respond to various objections in successive editions of their book; and their use of the principles is much more complex and nuanced, and extended by many more complementary considerations, than we can discuss here. But even those who reject this framework need to be familiar with it in order to understand how it is being employed within professional ethical discussions. We will be unable to take part in these important discussions unless we can understand the language and assumptions of others taking part – not least others who are advancing views that we believe need to be criticised. And more positively, the four principles do, many of us believe, offer some very useful – if limited – tools to help us to work towards ethical clarity.

Where do these principles come from? How might it be shown that they are ethically correct principles? Beauchamp and Childress claim that the principles can be derived from what they call "the common morality" – that is, from the morality common to the whole of humanity. They are appealing to what I have called our common moral sense. And it is very plausible to suggest that decent people from all places at all times would be able to recognise these as correct principles – certainly as principles that would correctly govern how one acts within particular contexts, such as within a caring relationship.[2] But it could also be argued that these principles can be supported by the different kinds of theories we have reviewed in the previous chapter. So a philosopher of a deontological persuasion might plausibly argue that these are *intrinsically* correct principles; that they tell us about certain general *duties* that we possess (the duty to act for the good of others, the duty to avoid harm to others, and so on). Such a philosopher might also claim that people (or at least our patients or clients and those affected by our work) have *rights* to be treated benevolently, and non-malevolently, and with respect for their autonomy, and justly. On the other hand, the consequentialist could argue – also with some plausibility – that it is by observing these principles that we will achieve the overall best *outcomes* for everyone concerned. And the rule utilitarian, in particular, could claim that these principles provide the rules that we should follow in order to bring about the greatest good. (Though I have argued that rule utilitarianism in particular, and consequentialism in general, should be rejected.) And the philosopher who concentrates on the virtues might readily accept that the virtuous person will be committed to these principles and will display that commitment in his or her traits of character.

Limitations of this framework

Beauchamp and Childress stress that as a framework for professional ethics, these principles are *limited* in two very important ways. First, the four principles do not display the whole extent of ethics – even of the ethics of the biomedical professions. They need to be, and can be, supplemented in various ways (e.g., by a concentration upon the required virtues of the professional person) if ethics is to be adequately described. And there are some very important ethical questions on which these principles may provide little help – or not the kind of help we most need. Think, for instance, of questions about how we ought to act towards a human embryo; or towards a rat or a baboon in a laboratory; or towards a patient who can no longer be restored to any level of consciousness. And think of questions about the extent to which we might engage in genetic engineering and other forms of human enhancement. These and other such questions bring us up against very deep philosophical issues at the foundations of professional ethics: to what sorts of thing do we have duties of care, and why? Why do we have particular duties of care towards the human person? What is the nature of this human person? What is the meaning and destiny of human life? And what does this imply about the nature and limits of our duties towards the human person? And so on. We will be considering some of these questions in our later chapters, and we will see that the four principles give us little, if any, help there.

The second important way in which the principles are limited is this. Even in the contexts in which they do apply, the four principles are limited in what they can show us about how we ought to act. They *do not provide a formula for action.* They are too *general* to do that. They do not tell us specifically what to do, but they do state an essential norm or value that must always be respected. They provide *very general guidelines* for our conduct. However, more specific rules can be derived from the principles, as we shall see by considering each principle in turn.

Spelling out the principles

The principle of ***beneficence*** has a very natural place within the service or caring professions. Medicine, nursing, social work and other such professions are *essentially committed* to the *good*, the welfare, of the people they serve. That commitment is the *raison d'être* of the profession. It may be difficult in particular cases to identify what would *be* good for some patient or client; but there need be no question that the professional ought to be acting for that good, whatever it is. And training in the profession essentially consists in learning, in a wide variety of particular ways, what would be good and how that good is to be brought about. (What ailment are we presented with here? What would be its remedy? How is that remedy to be achieved? What is bad about this situation and how can we assist to improve it? And so on.) These professionals learn the specific rules derived from the principle of beneficence by learning the skills of their profession.

The principle of ***non-maleficence*** has a similarly obvious place within the serving professions. If our purpose is to act for the good, then we clearly need to avoid causing what is bad. Nevertheless, as we shall see, there is a point in keeping the principle of non-maleficence distinct from the principle of beneficence rather than regarding them as merely two aspects of one principle. Traditionally, the principle of non-maleficence was sometimes *spoken of* as if it were the dominant principle: "*first*, do no harm" was the commonly expressed rule. But that slogan made sense *within* a medical context in which there was *already* a commitment to the good of the patient and in which it was very important to remember that one's attempts to do good must avoid doing harm. It would be a mistake, however, as we shall also see, to think that the principle of non-maleficence is always of *overriding* importance. If the most important moral rule were that we must always avoid doing harm, then there would be a very simple way to obey it – by doing nothing at all! And this, of course, would defeat the very purpose of the caring professions. So the principle of non-maleficence operates *alongside* the principle of beneficence; and members learn the many very specific ways in which they need to obey it as they learn the skills of their profession. (What damage could we do here? What are the risks and possible side-effects of this or that treatment or intervention? How probable are they, and how harmful would they be? How are they to be weighed against the good that we would do? How, precisely, is this or that damage to be avoided? And so on.)

Sometimes students are a little confused about what the principles of beneficence and non-maleficence are referring to. Because professional care is often a matter of intervening to repair some *harm* that has occurred (through disease or accident, say, or through a bad social situation), the student might suppose that this professional intervention is an instance of following the principle of non-maleficence – that in intervening, the professional is avoiding harm. But that would be a misunderstanding of the kind of harm that this principle is referring to. The principle of non-maleficence is concerned with *harm that the professional could do*; it is *this* harm that it instructs us to avoid. When a doctor acts to cure a disease or a social worker makes arrangements in order to improve a bad situation, each is trying to repair harm, but not harm that they have caused. Each, in trying to repair this harm, is *acting for the good*. So each is following the principle of *beneficence*. And of course, an enormous amount of the good done by the service and caring professions consists in action to repair some harm that has occurred naturally or by accident or through the harmful doings of other persons.

The principle of ***autonomy*** has become more prominent in the ethics of the caring professions over recent decades. Beauchamp and Childress help us to see what it can mean in practice by arguing that there is a cluster of more specific rules which fall within its scope. From the principle of autonomy, we can derive rules concerning the need for informed consent for treatment; for truth-telling; for respect for privacy and confidentiality; and for various kinds of assistance in decision-making. What is the connection between these matters and autonomy? When patients or clients are autonomous, they have the liberty and the ability to determine what is done to them. And their determining what is done to them of course requires that they consent to what is done. If their consent is to be genuine, it must not be coerced or manipulated. And if it is to be real consent *to* what is actually going to happen, it needs to be properly informed. The patient or client needs to be supplied with the information that he or she requires in order to be able to make a good choice between the various possible options. This in turn requires that the professional tells the truth. But even when armed with the truth, the patient or client might still require assistance and emotional support in order to appreciate the various options and their possible consequences, and to face them clearly in thinking about them and weighing them appropriately. So the professional needs to be ready to offer this assistance and support.

But what does autonomy have to do with privacy and confidentiality? Matters which are private are those that we wish not to make public, or that others should expect that we may wish not to make public. We can choose to reveal or disclose these matters to some other person (to someone intimate with us, for instance; or to someone who needs to know those matters if they are to act on our behalf). But in doing this, we are not revealing these matters to the rest of the world. Rather, we are trusting that person – *confiding* in that person – to preserve the privacy of what we reveal. Unless, of course, we give that person *permission* to reveal those matters more generally. But it is *up to us* to determine who has access to those matters. In other words, it is an aspect of our proper autonomy, our governing what happens to us, that *we* determine who has access to our private concerns. And this requires the professional who does have access to our private matters to protect the privacy of those matters – to ensure that others do not have access to our private body, or to our private activities, or to our private documents, or to the information that we have confided to him or her. It is not for the professional to determine who has access to these things; it is for us to decide.

The requirements of the principle of ***justice*** can be easily *stated*: we ought to act justly. It is much less easy, however, to spell out all that this means in detail. There is a huge amount of philosophical discussion and debate about the various details of the requirements of justice. But our ordinary working notions of justice can take us a long way in working out what is just or unjust in some practical situation. In the context of professional service, it is convenient to think of the first three principles as focused upon our relation to our client or patient. Thus, we are required by those principles to act for the good of the client, to avoid harm to the client, and to respect the autonomy of the client. But the principle of justice reminds us that how we act towards our client may also affect other people – third parties. And it directs us to ensure that the way we act towards our client is not unjust towards those other people. We must ensure that the interests of those other people – their good, their need not to be harmed, their autonomy – are also appropriately protected. (We shall see some examples of this shortly.) Our direct professional duty may be to our client, but we must not act towards our client in a way that is unjust towards others. (And if we have more than one client, then of course justice will require that we act justly towards them all, as well as towards third parties – people who are not our clients.)

Relations between the principles

How are these principles related to one another? This is a very pressing question whenever there is more than one moral principle that applies to a particular situation – for, given that the principles are different, they could guide us in different practical directions, and in that case we will need to know more than simply what the principles say if we are to know what direction to follow. Take a classic kind of case often discussed. Suppose that there is a moral principle that we ought to tell the truth, and another moral principle that we ought not to expose innocent people to unjust attack. And suppose that we know the whereabouts of some innocent person who is being pursued by a powerful and wicked enemy. That enemy apprehends us and demands to know the whereabouts of the innocent person. Here the requirements of the two principles clash with one another: to tell the truth would be to expose the innocent person to an unjust attack; but to protect the innocent person would require us to breach our duty to tell the truth (by keeping silent, or – and this may be the only effective way to protect the person – by lying to the enemy). How are we to act? The important thing to see here is that we cannot answer this question merely by looking at what the principles tell us to do. We need to know more than that: we need to know which principle is the most important one – or at least which principle is concerned with what morally matters most in this particular case. Which is the principle of overriding importance? Our decision-making would become straightforward if we knew that the principles were so related to one another that they formed a *hierarchy* – that Principle 1 is always more important than Principle 2 (that when these two principles clash, Principle 1 always *overrides* or *trumps* Principle 2), and that Principle 2 is always more important than Principle 3, and so on. Knowing the hierarchy would then enable us to know which principle to follow in the situation where two or more principles clash. But Beauchamp and Childress argue that the four principles do *not* form a hierarchy: no principle is always more important than any of the others. For each principle, there will be certain situations in which it is the most important principle, but other situations in which its claims are overridden by one or more of the other principles. This means that the principles are *prima facie* principles: each one tells us what to do "at first sight"; each gives us a reason to act in a particular way, but this reason could be overridden by other reasons. Each principle makes a moral claim which ought to be obeyed *other things being equal.* But there will be situations in which other things won't be equal – in which other principles also make moral claims, and their claims, in those situations, have a greater moral force.

Philosophers particularly enjoy discussing cases in which two or more ethical principles clash with each other. Typically, these cases are *hard* cases, and hard cases are especially interesting cases. But what makes them interesting is not simply the fact that they provide good intellectual sport. They are interesting because in thinking about these cases, we may better understand the relative *scope and significance* of each of the principles concerned. As we reflect upon the cases we may feel, for instance, that Principle 1 is the overridingly important principle in *this* case, but that Principle 2 is the overridingly important principle in *that* case. But then we will be in a position to work away at such questions as: what is it about *this* case that shows that it falls within the area dominated by Principle 1; and what is it about *that* case that shows that it falls within the bounds of the dominance of Principle 2; and what does all of that tell us about what each principle is getting at, about how important that is, and about how far it extends? The difficult cases are the ones that help us to recognise the limits of each principle in relation to the limits of the other principles.

Applying the principles: easy cases

The four principles will show that there are many such hard cases in professional ethics, and we will look at some of those shortly. But before we do that, we can note that it would be foolish to suppose that the principles never give us perfectly straightforward, clear moral guidance. Many cases are not hard cases at all, and the principles show us why they are not. Indeed, probably the greater proportion of our professional service will involve work within cases in which our ethical duties, as defined by the principles, are quite clear. So for instance, imagine that some doctor does something that causes some unjustified harm to her patient, and that she does this simply because she is indifferent to the patient's wellbeing; or because she is inadequately diligent; or because she hasn't properly acquired the relevant skills or has let them get rusty; or because she hasn't kept up with the necessary ongoing training; or because she is over-treating the patient (because of bad judgement, or a wrong fear of legal consequences, or through a greedy wish to charge higher fees); or because she is impaired (by disease, or alcohol, or drugs…). In any of these situations, the doctor would have acted in a way that is clearly ethically wrong: she would have breached the principle of non-maleficence.

Or imagine that a doctor fails to do some good that he ought to do for his patient because he is indifferent or inadequately diligent or negligently under-skilled; or because he is under-treating the patient; or because he abandons the care of the patient without ensuring adequate replacement care; or because he neglects to educate the patient about what lies ahead or to provide proper preventive care… These are all situations in which the doctor would clearly have breached the principle of beneficence.

Or imagine a case in which a doctor fails to get her patient's clear, properly informed consent for treatment because she is indifferent; or because she negligently forgets to do so; or because she does not tell the patient the truth, or enough of the truth, about his situation; or because what she tells the patient cannot be understood by him; or because she does not give him proper time to deliberate and decide; or because his decision is coerced (by the doctor, or by others of whom the doctor should be aware); or because his decision is manipulated (by the doctor or others). Or imagine that the doctor gives herself unjustified access to private information about the patient – information to which she has no right as part of her care for him. Or imagine that the doctor gives herself unjustified access to the private goings-on of the patient (when he is undressed, perhaps, or otherwise requiring privacy) – access to which she has no right as part of her care for him. Or imagine that she leaves the patient in conditions where other people have unjustified access to his private goings-on. Or imagine that the doctor provides confidential information about the patient to some other person – a person who has no proper claim to that information through his responsibility of care for, or relationship with, the patient. These would all be clear wrongs: they would all be breaches of the principle of respect for the patient's autonomy.

Or imagine that a doctor treats his patient in such a way that *another* patient cannot be treated in a way that *he* is entitled to (because the doctor spends an unfair amount of time, or an unfair amount of the available medical resources, on the first patient). Or imagine that the doctor distributes his treatment unfairly because he distributes it according to irrelevant criteria (he gives priority, or more adequate treatment, to patients of a particular race, or social status…). Or imagine that he treats his patients in such a way that it imposes an unfair burden upon others (e.g., members of a medical aid scheme, or taxpayers). These would all clearly be wrongs: they would be breaches of the principle of justice.

So we see that there are many cases in which there need be no ethical confusion or unclarity. We may not need to have *heard* of the four principles to recognise the wrongs we have just imagined. But the four principles can describe for us *why* they are wrongs. And it is easy to see how the kinds of cases that we have just imagined could be changed into cases involving not a doctor, but a social worker or another member of the caring professions.

Various kinds of hard case

Nevertheless, the kinds of cases in which it is easy – at least for the uninvolved onlooker – to *describe* what is ethically correct may not be cases in which it is easy to *do* what is ethically correct. Some hard cases are hard not because it is hard to *know* what to do, but because it is hard to *do* it. The professional may be under some pressure to act in an ethically compromised or indeed in a thoroughly wrong way. He may be under pressure from the organisation within which he works, or from his social group, or from his own powerful temptations to cut corners or to make money. In such a case proper action is not guaranteed simply through knowledge of the relevant ethical principles. What is required is a very firm *commitment* to those principles, and mere awareness of the principles is not enough to ensure that commitment. Even so, given our propensity to deceive ourselves in order to rationalise the wrongs that we wish to do, we can at least make it easier for ourselves to maintain our ethical commitments by *reflecting upon* the principles – by turning our mind to them and to their importance; by keeping our minds ethically clear rather than surrendering to a fog of self-deceptive rationalisation. And a clear-headed commitment to the principles is something which professionals, and those close to them, can *encourage* in one another.

But let us turn now to ethically hard cases that are hard because it is hard to *know* what to do. Many of these, as we have said, are cases in which two or more principles clash. But not all of the hard cases are of that kind. Imagine that you are in charge of the neo-natal intensive care unit of a hospital, and two premature babies – both delivered this morning – are brought up to you for intensive care. Each is likely to die without a place in your unit. But there is only one place available (and no other places within travelling distance). What are you to do? Do you allocate the available place on a "first come, first served" basis? But what if the two babies have been brought up to your unit together? Do you give the place to the baby who needs it more? But what if they are equally likely to die unless they receive the place? Or what if the baby who is slightly less likely to die *without* the place is also slightly more likely to live if *given* the place? Would it make a difference if one of the babies, but not the other, was disabled; or if one of the babies, but not the other, had two loving and committed parents? Should *any* of those considerations be regarded as relevant? Can it be said that each baby has the same right to your best care and that you should therefore allocate the place by tossing a coin or by using some other "lottery" procedure…? These are agonisingly difficult questions. They arise not because there is a clash between the different principles, but because it is extraordinarily difficult to know what the one relevant principle requires of us in such a case. These are questions about what the *principle of justice* requires. What is the just way to distribute limited resources? A vast amount has been said in response to this question, and in response to other hard questions concerning what a particular principle requires in a certain kind of case. But it would be foolish to suppose that the answers are easy or obvious.

Applying the principles when they clash with one another

We come now to the cases in which two or more principles clash. Beauchamp and Childress claim that each of the four principles is only a *prima facie* principle, and so that there will be a full range of the possible situations in which one principle overrides another. We can display this by using the grid set out in Figure 5.1. What does the grid mean? Each column of the grid has a principle stated at its head, and each row of the grid has a principle stated at its side. A section of the grid contains any situation – any possible case – in which the requirements of the principle at the top of the column override, or outweigh or trump, the requirements of the principle in the row. So, for instance, the section I have marked as B/N is for cases in which the requirements of the principle of beneficence outweigh the requirements of the principle of non-maleficence; whereas the section marked as N/B is for cases in which the converse is true (non-maleficence trumps beneficence). If each principle is *prima facie*, if no principle is always more important than any other principle, then for each section of the grid, we would expect to be able to find possible cases which properly belong within that section. (The shaded sections cannot contain any case, for there cannot be a case where the requirements of a principle override *themselves*.)

	Beneficence	Non-maleficence	Autonomy	Justice
Beneficence		N/B	A/B	J/B
Non-maleficence	B/N		A/N	J/N
Autonomy	B/A	N/A		J/A
Justice	B/J	N/J	A/J	

Figure 5.1

But how do we identify the section to which a case properly belongs? If a case is one to which two principles apply, but their requirements clash with one another, how are we to work out which one is the overriding principle? Earlier I discussed how hard cases may help us to see the limits of the various principles, and what I said there took for granted that we may be able to work out the relative weights of the two principles as we think about the cases. I said that as we reflect on one case, we may feel that Principle 1 overrides the importance of Principle 2 in that case, but that in another case it is the other way around. Now we would be unable to reach such judgements if we did not possess our own *moral sense* that allows us to weigh the importance of the two principles in the different cases. If all we have is the principles themselves, then we have nothing by which we can weigh them. We need some independent measure if we are to judge their relative weights. And this is what is provided by our intuitive moral sense – the common moral sense to which I have repeatedly referred. That is not to say that our moral sense is so clear that we will always to be able to reach a definite decision about the case. But nor do we need to despair of making progress. Beauchamp and Childress believe that our method should be that of the *reflective equilibrium* which we have referred to in previous chapters. Through thoughtful, sensitive reflection upon each case, consulting our own moral intuitions, we should seek to discern the right balance between the claims of the different principles. (Beauchamp and Childress believe that we should also consult what various moral theories might say, and any other relevant contributions to the ethical discussion, and should reflect about where the right overall balance is to be found given all these considerations. But at the moment, let us keep our task relatively straightforward by concentrating simply upon the balance between the four principles and our own intuitions about a case.)

Let us see how this can work by performing a series of exercises in which we review a range of particular cases. Many of the cases that will most clearly show how two principles clash are cases that occur within the healthcare arena – the arena in which the four principles have been put to the most work within the academic discussion. But we will also consider some distinctive social work cases, to see how the four-principles framework applies there. The healthcare cases are not, of course, of mere theoretical interest to those in social work, social welfare and so on, for much of the professional work in these fields overlaps with healthcare. Many of those who work in the wider caring professions will find themselves involved in healthcare cases such as those we will review below.

But before we look at my cases, I invite the reader to perform his or her own preliminary exercise. I suggest that, for each section of the grid in Figure 5.1, you try to think of some actual situation in professional practice that properly fits within that section. Thus, for section B/N, you should think of a situation in which both the principle of beneficence and the principle of non-maleficence do apply, but the requirements of the principle of beneficence outweigh those of the principle of non-maleficence. For section N/B, you should think of a situation where both those principles apply, but the outweighing principle is the principle of non-maleficence. And so on for all the other sections. Try to think of as many different cases as you can for each section. I suggest that you do this before reading any further, for I think that you will profit more by what we are going on to discuss if you have already performed this little exercise.

Presuming, now, that you *have* spent some time on that exercise, let's make some observations about it. Many students get stuck on Section B/N of the grid: they find it very hard to think of some real situation in which the requirements of beneficence override those of non-maleficence. But that is because they are trying to think of something unusual. In fact, virtually *every* case of proper medical treatment, or indeed of proper healthcare treatment, belongs in this section. Consider this utterly usual case. A doctor properly prescribes medication for a patient. But that medication has some actual side-effects which are not very serious (perhaps it makes the patient drowsy), and some possible side-effects which would be serious but are very unlikely (perhaps it could cause a severe allergic reaction). Those side-effects would be *harmful*, and the principle of non-maleficence requires the doctor to avoid that actual or possible harm. Does that mean that the doctor is doing the wrong thing in prescribing that medication? Of course not, because the *good* that the doctor is seeking to do in curing or relieving the patient's ailment is important enough to outweigh the severity of the actual harm plus the risk of the serious harm. Beneficence here trumps non-maleficence. But of course, the doctor would be *unjustified* in prescribing that medicine unless it were for that important good purpose (which is why such medicines are not available over the counter). Unless the principle of beneficence *did* apply, the principle of non-maleficence *would* forbid the prescription of the medicine. In surgical cases, this relation between the two principles is even more obvious. Surgical invasion of the body is certainly harmful. (No surgeon, or anyone else, is entitled to wield a scalpel willy-nilly!) But the doing of that harm can be justified *so long as* the good that one is seeking to do is important and probable enough to outweigh the harm done. And so on throughout the healthcare professions, for virtually every kind of treatment carries some risks or harmful burdens, but is aimed at some worthwhile good that outweighs the burdens and risks. (Think about the pain that can be caused by the physiotherapist. And many of us would prefer *not* to think about going to the dentist…)

And Section N/B is for cases in which the relation is the other way around. There are many cases in which the normal treatment that a healthcare professional would seek to use in order to perform some important good – the treatment that the principle of beneficence would normally require – would in this particular case cause such a burden of harm, or such a risk of serious harm, that it would be unjustified to use that treatment. The requirements of the principle of non-maleficence here trump those of the principle of beneficence. (There may be reason to suppose that a particular patient has a *high* risk of a very severe allergic reaction. Or think, for instance, of a case in which a frail, very elderly patient has advanced cancer. Very invasive surgery plus chemotherapy and radiotherapy may manage to extend the patient's life by some months. But the burden of pain and discomfort and distress that this would cause may well be so great as to outweigh the good that it could do.)

In thinking about those two sections of the grid, we *have* been able to see where some cases fit. We have been able, in other words, to see how the right balance is to be struck between the two principles that apply to the case. Our moral sense has been able to do that work for us. And you might have been able to do similar work in finding the right balance within the other pairs of principles, in imagining cases which fit in the other sections of the grid. But we are now going to consider a list of particular cases for that purpose. And if you have already imagined cases, you can compare your cases with those which we are about to consider.

As you read each case in the list below, I invite you to do your best to work out where it fits on the grid in Figure 5.1. Again, it will help to do this before you read what I say in reviewing the case. I am inviting you, in other words, to identify the principles that apply to the case, and to work out the right balance between the claims of those principles – thereby identifying the section of the grid in which the case fits. You are, of course, asking what the professional ought to do in the case. In many of the cases, the professional involved faces a choice between different courses of action. In these cases, you should ask what choice the professional ought to make, and why. In some of the cases, the professional has already made a particular choice. In those cases, you should be asking whether the choice was right or wrong, and why; and if it was wrong, you will be identifying the section of the grid into which the right choice would have fitted. Don't be surprised if this is difficult in some of the cases. (Some of them are cases in which it ought to be difficult.) If you struggle with a case, at least do your best to answer the following questions: what further information about the case might assist you to determine where the case belongs? If a certain choice in this case *would be* the right choice, where on the grid would the case belong? But if that choice would be the wrong choice, where on the grid would the case belong?

Case 1

Dr P, a GP, is engaged in an appointment with Mrs Q, a dear old lady who, in her faltering and rather ill-focused and long-winded fashion, is expressing her anxieties about a number of complicated medical concerns. Dr P knows that she could genuinely help Mrs Q if she spent more time discussing those concerns. But she ends the appointment. There is a queue in the waiting room.

Case 2

A young man needs surgery for a serious condition. This need is thoroughly explained to him, and he discusses it carefully with the medical team. There is no good alternative treatment. He refuses to undergo the surgery.

Case 3

A man arrives in the casualty department of a large public hospital on a Saturday night. He has been involved in a fight and urgently requires surgery. He is drunk and confused, and conscious only some of the time. During his periods of consciousness, he loudly protests that he doesn't want to be treated, but wants to be allowed to go home *now*.

Case 4

A passenger on a flight from western Africa disembarks with signs of a fever. The authorities order that he be placed in quarantine.

Case 5

Dr R is a GP. One of her patients, Mr S, has returned a positive result to an HIV test. Dr R carefully counsels Mr S, and alerts him to the need to inform his wife. But Mr S insists that his wife must not be told.

Case 6

A 13-year-old girl, unconscious after a car accident, is brought into the hospital's casualty department by her extremely worried parents. She desperately needs a blood transfusion. But the parents refuse consent: they are Jehovah's Witnesses (and thus, on religious grounds, conscientiously object to blood transfusion). Furthermore, they say that their daughter would also refuse consent.

Case 7

Betty is a childless 26-year-old woman who has returned a positive result to a pap smear test (for cervical cancer). Her GP, Dr K, refers Betty to the oncologist, Dr H. But Dr K finds out later that Betty did not go to see Dr H. Dr K knows that the cancer risk ought to be investigated swiftly. He tries to telephone Betty, but gets no answer. So he telephones Betty's husband Dan, alerting him to the possibility of cancer and asking him to urge Betty to go to see Dr H.[3]

Case 8

Betty does go to see Dr H. Stage 1 cancer is diagnosed; radiation therapy is advised, and with radiotherapy, the prognosis is good. Betty studies the literature, and demands instead a radical hysterectomy, on the ground that this will ensure that the problem is dealt with. Dr H believes that a hysterectomy is not required.[4]

Case 9

Dr X has a rather neurotically anxious patient, Mr Y, who is troubled by insomnia. Mr Y asks for sleeping pills. Dr X gives Mr Y some tablets, telling him that he is sure that they will help. Mr Y later reports that the tablets have done him a lot of good, and he is now sleeping much better. The tablets are a placebo.

Case 10

A doctor in a remote rural area has just performed an extremely difficult delivery. The baby is dying, and the mother is critically ill. The mother desperately asks the doctor, "How is my baby?" The doctor knows from bitter experience that if he tells the mother the truth, she may well turn her face to the wall and give up and die; but if she believes that there is hope for her baby, she may well fight on and live.

Case 11

Many patients who die of kidney failure could be saved by a kidney transplant, but there are far too few donor kidneys for the required number of transplants. Most of us have two kidneys, and could do without one of them. The national health authority is considering two proposals which would save the lives of many kidney-disease patients. The first proposal is that kidneys should be surgically removed, *post mortem*, from all road accident patients who die under emergency care, whether or not these patients have consented to the donation of their kidneys. One disadvantage of this proposal is that it may not produce enough donor kidneys to save the lives of all the kidney-disease patients. This is not a disadvantage shared by the second proposal, which is that there should be a system of compulsory national service in *live* kidney donation: healthy donors would be selected by lottery, and those selected would be required to have a kidney surgically removed. A sufficient number of donor kidneys would thereby be made available.

Case 12

Some of the public hospitals within the main city of a developing country have fine neo-natal intensive care units (ICUs). These hospitals have a policy of not admitting to these units babies with a birth weight less than 1,000 grams (gm), even though the units could care for premature babies with birth weights of very much less than this. The reason for this policy is that many more premature babies are born than can be cared for using the limited facilities across the hospitals. On a busy Saturday night, an intern delivers a premature baby with a birth weight of 840gm. Uncertain about what is expected of her, the intern places the baby under the intensive care that it needs. When he arrives for work on Monday morning, the consultant in charge discovers this baby in the ICU. The baby is doing well.

Presuming, now, that you have done your own thinking about where these cases fit on the grid, let us work over each one in turn. As we look at each case, I shall not try to provide a full resolution of it, but shall make some observations about how the four principles help us to clarify what is at stake. That, I hope, will allow you to think further about the case and work towards what you believe to be its correct resolution.

Case 1 involves the sort of situation that any caring professional is presented with nearly all the time. Dr P knows that there is more *good* that she can do for Mrs Q, but she ends the appointment because she doesn't want to be *unfair* to her other patients. She needs to distribute the limited resource of her time *justly*. So the clash here is between the requirements of the principle of beneficence and those of the principle of justice. And if she has acted correctly in ending the appointment, the case fits in section J/B of the grid – the section for the cases in which the requirements of the principle of justice override or trump the requirements of the principle of beneficence. But *has she* acted correctly? Was she right to end the appointment when she did? What further information might help you to answer that question? (For instance, how urgent and important were Mrs Q's further concerns? Were there other ways in which those concerns could have been properly attended to? How pressing were the needs of the waiting patients? If Dr P did need to end the appointment when she did, was there more that she could have done to ensure that she was ending the appointment in a way that cared properly for Mrs Q? And so on. And how might the answers to those questions indicate *the relative weights in this particular case* of what the principle of beneficence is concerned with, on the one hand, and what the principle of justice is concerned with, on the other?)

Case 2 presents a straightforward clash between what would be for the *good* of the patient, on the one hand, and what he *wants*, on the other. A patient is ethically entitled to refuse treatment, and if this is such a case then it belongs in section A/B of the grid – for cases in which the requirements of the principle of autonomy override those of the principle of beneficence. But no caring professional should find it easy to resolve such a case simply by dismissing the patient while saying, "Well, that's what he wants." The patient *needs* the treatment which he is refusing, and the caring professional will be very concerned if this need is not being met. The professional can at least do his best to find out *why* the young man is refusing treatment, and to deal with what emerges. (Sometimes treatment is refused for good reason. But sometimes it is refused because of misunderstanding, or misplaced fear, or depression, or a concern not to burden others…)

Like the previous case, **Case 3** presents a clash between what the patient wants and what is for his good – and thus between the requirements of the principle of autonomy and those of the principle of beneficence. But unlike the previous case, this one probably does not belong in section A/B of the grid. It belongs rather in section B/A, in which the requirements of beneficence trump those of autonomy – and is thus a case in which the patient ought to be treated despite his protests. (The doctors will know how to proceed. Some sedation may help.) An important difference between this case and Case 2 is that in this case, the patient's autonomy is *impaired*: his physical condition renders him unable to act as a fully autonomous person – as a person who has the freedom and the capacity to make properly judged decisions about what should be done to him. And thus his actual wants at the moment have a much lower significance than his actual needs. Furthermore, in treating him for his *good*, the hospital team are also seeking to restore him to a condition in which he can again function as a properly autonomous individual. A related way to think about the situation is to ask not what the patient *does* want now, but what he *would* want if he were considering the situation he is in now from a properly rational perspective; and surely the hospital team could be entitled to believe that if this were the case, then he would want to be treated. And thus, though beneficence here outweighs autonomy insofar as the patient's good is more important than what he *actually* wants, it does not outweigh it in regard to what he *would properly* want. Rather, his good and his *proper* autonomy *coincide* in what they require. Emergency medicine, of course, faces cases like this all the time.

The person placed in quarantine in **Case 4** is deprived of his liberty in various ways, and thus his autonomy is interfered with (because he is not free to determine what happens to him). He is also probably harmed in some ways (because he is unable to see his family, or do his paid work, and so on). So his being placed under quarantine is contrary to the *prima facie* principles of autonomy and non-maleficence. Nevertheless, his confinement will be justified if he, in his diseased condition, presents a serious threat to the health of others, in which case the requirements of the principle of justice will outweigh those of the principles of autonomy and non-maleficence. And so such a case belongs to sections J/A and J/N of the grid. (It might be thought that his being quarantined is also for his own good, and so required by the principle of beneficence. But this is probably a mistake, for though the authorities should be trying to cure him, it is unlikely that he needs to be *quarantined* in order for his disease to be treated.) And even though the principles of autonomy and non-maleficence are overridden in these cases, the authorities, while ensuring that public health is protected, will, if they are acting properly, also ensure that the patient is deprived of his liberty no more than and for no longer than is necessary, and that harm to him is avoided in any way possible. In other words, the principles of autonomy and non-maleficence are still *applicable* to the case, even though they are not overriding. Many cases involving quarantine orders do of course fit in this way in sections J/A and J/N of the grid. But does Case 4? Do the facts before us show that this is a *justified* quarantine order? A quarantine order could, of course, be unjustified – because the patient does not present a genuine threat to public health, or because the order is malicious, or in some other way.

What further facts would you need to know before you could determine whether the authorities' order was ethically correct?

In **Case 5**, Dr R knows that Mr S's infection seriously endangers the health – indeed perhaps the life – of Mrs S (presuming, as Dr R may have every reason to presume, that Mr S intends to continue to have ordinary sexual relations with Mrs S). But it is clear that Mr S does not intend to inform his wife of his infection, and it would certainly be a very serious matter for Dr R to inform Mrs S. Dr R's doing this would constitute a serious breach of confidentiality, and it may cause considerable harm in disturbing Mr S's relationship with Mrs S; and thus it would be opposed by both autonomy and non-maleficence. Nevertheless, as I have argued elsewhere,[5] Dr R may well be justified in taking action to inform Mrs S. There are cases in which a doctor is *obliged* to warn some identifiable third party of a threat posed to them by the patient, because what is at stake for this third party (the concern of justice) is so grave as to outweigh the importance of the patient's autonomy and protection from harm. Such a case would therefore belong, as Case 4 could belong, to sections J/A and J/N of the grid. But once again, in taking proper action to inform Mrs S, Dr R would try to *limit* the breach of confidentiality and the harm that it could cause. How might she try to do that?

In **Case 6**, the hospital team will be earnestly attempting to give the 13-year-old girl the blood transfusion on which her life may well depend. They will be seeking to act for her *good*. Because she is unconscious, she cannot consent to this treatment. But, as in so many other cases of emergency medicine (e.g., Case 3), the fact that there is no consent is insufficient to prevent the hospital team from acting for her good, because the requirements of the principle of beneficence are here weighty enough to trump those of the principle of autonomy, which normally include the need for consent. However, because the girl is a minor, her parents have a proper moral authority to act on her behalf; and they refuse consent. Furthermore, they say that she herself would refuse consent (and we may have no reason to doubt that they are telling the truth). And at 13 years old, the girl is nearing the age when we should attach as much significance to what she wants as we would to what an adult wants. So is this case more like Case 2 than Case 3? Is it a case where the requirements of the principle of autonomy override those of beneficence – a case which belongs to section A/B of the grid, in which the hospital team ought not to perform the transfusion?

The hospital team would rightly be troubled by that suggestion. The refusal of consent is here grounded in religious conviction, and the principle of autonomy properly insists that we take people's religious convictions very seriously. Someone's religious convictions can be at the heart of who he is as a person;

and when we make him act or be acted upon in a way that is inconsistent with those convictions, we can be attacking his very core. But a life-threatening illness is also an attack upon his very person; and if we know that his religious convictions prevent us from saving his life, then we may have powerful reason to believe that, though it would be bad to override what he wants, it would be even worse to have our action on his behalf constrained by those convictions. This is especially true if we have reason to suspect that his refusal of treatment could perhaps change, or that it is driven by convictions which are not of absolute importance to him. (Interestingly enough, some doctors have testified that when they provide life-saving treatment to someone who has on principle refused, or would refuse, the treatment, the patient shows after recovery that they are glad that the treatment was provided. The patient may have felt honour-bound to refuse the treatment, but is glad that this refusal was overridden, and that the doctor accepted the responsibility to act.)

But beneficence speaks all the more powerfully against autonomy when it is a child's life at stake. A 13-year-old girl is advancing in maturity, but we do not regard her as having yet attained the age when she can enjoy a properly mature autonomy in relation to the deepest and most irrevocable decisions concerning life and death; so her own refusal of life-saving treatment, even if correctly reported by her parents, cannot be weighty enough to stop us saving her life. What about the refusal by her parents? Parents do have a proper authority to speak on behalf of their children. But this authority derives in part from the fact that we presume that the parent is able to assess what is in the best interests of the child, and is acting in those interests. And this presumption can be overturned. Where we have proper reason to believe that the parent is not recognising or not acting in the best interests of the child, we can, in some sufficiently weighty matter (e.g., the life or death of the child), act in those interests ourselves in a way which overrides the parent's authority. These are reasons for the hospital team to judge that Case 6 belongs in section B/A of the grid, where beneficence outweighs autonomy – and that they ought to perform the blood transfusion. In many countries the law helps them to do so. (And it could perhaps turn out afterwards that the parents are grateful.)

In **Case 7**, Dr K is very concerned to act in a way that protects Betty's health. He knows that there is some urgency, for if cancer is the correct diagnosis, then early treatment is very important. He cannot wait indefinitely for Betty to see the oncologist. He is acting for Betty's good, as required by the principle of beneficence. But in order to do this, he has informed a third party of Betty's test result and the possible danger to her health, and he has done so without Betty's consent. He has breached confidentiality, and thus the principle of autonomy. In discussing Case 5, we saw how breach of a patient's confidentiality might be justified by the need to act for the good of some third party, and thus by the requirements of justice. But in Case 7, Dr K is breaching confidentiality for the patient's own good. Is this an unjustified violation of the principle of autonomy? If it is, then he ought not to have contacted Dan, Betty's husband, in the way he did, and the case properly belongs to section A/B of the grid, where the requirements of autonomy override those of beneficence. But if he was right to contact Dan, then the case belongs to section B/A, where the requirements of autonomy are overridden by those of beneficence. Was he right?

Dr K has not informed just anyone of Betty's test result. He has told her husband, who, we would hope, would be at least as concerned for Betty's health and the protection of her confidentiality as is Dr K, and would be trusted – confided in – by Betty at least as much as she confides in Dr K. Because of this very proper closeness between patient and family members, and because of the family members' deep concern to protect and act for the welfare of the patient, it is often thoroughly appropriate to enlist the support of the family members in patient care and to ensure that they understand enough of the patient's situation to be able to offer effective help. But of course, a family situation can be less than ideal. We may be in a situation where the family members cannot be presumed to be acting in the best interests of our patient or client, or where we cannot presume that the patient would be prepared to confide in some family member; and in any such situation, the breach of confidentiality could be seriously wrong. Might Dr K have known enough about Betty and Dan's situation to have been justified in telephoning Dan? Could further information help you to evaluate Dr K's action? Or was the urgent need to be acting to protect Betty's health sufficient to justify his action?

Case 8 concerns the next step in Betty's medical history. It is another case which helps us to test the limits of the principle of autonomy. Betty – who is only 26 – is demanding a radical hysterectomy. The oncologist, Dr H, does not believe that this would be the appropriate treatment. She knows that a much more conservative treatment, radiotherapy, is likely to deal with the cancer; whereas a hysterectomy would entail all the harm of major surgery and would remove one of Betty's very important organs, rendering her unable to bear children. In other words, Dr H believes that a hysterectomy would be more harmful than is required. We can suppose, of course, that she properly discusses all of this with Betty. But Betty continues to insist upon the hysterectomy: she wants this cancer scare put behind her in the most decisive way. Should Dr H accede to Betty's demand, or is this a case in which she ought not to be governed by what Betty wants because here the requirements of non-maleficence override those of autonomy? Does this case belong to section A/N or to section N/A of the grid?

There surely are various kinds of case in which our duty not to do harm to a patient trumps our duty to do as the patient wants. A woman who feels that she would be more beautiful if she had a perfectly healthy arm removed is not entitled to insist that we perform the amputation, even if she is of sound mind (at least in any of the *other* respects that display her mental condition). We typically do not believe that it is right to give a lethal injection to a patient who feels that his life is not worth living. Rather, we believe that our duty is to provide proper supportive care for him – the very care which might, as things turn out, cause him to alter his own assessment of the value of his life. So it seems that we accept that there is an asymmetry between what a patient is entitled to *demand* in the way of positive treatment, on the one hand, and what he is entitled to *refuse*, on the other. In discussing Case 2, we imagined situations in which a medical team, while seeking to provide very important – perhaps life-saving – treatment, might sadly have to accede to a patient's refusal of that treatment. But now we are discussing the fact that a medical team does not have to accede to a patient's demand for unnecessarily harmful treatment. Thus the principle of autonomy is more powerful where it applies to the patient's refusal of treatment than where it applies to the patient's demand for treatment. And Betty's demand for a hysterectomy – insofar as it is a demand for what is unnecessarily harmful – seems to fall beyond the proper limit of the principle of autonomy.

Someone might protest that it is *up to Betty* to decide whether the hysterectomy would be unnecessarily harmful. *We* might say that it is unnecessarily harmful because it will prevent her from ever having children. But in stating her demand for the hysterectomy, Betty is showing that she does *not want* to have children. So she does not assess this as undue harm – and who are we to impose our assessment over hers? The protester is, of course, correct to claim that it is up to Betty whether she has children. But we all know that our wishes on these matters can change over time. (There are many women in their 30s who are glad that they are still able to have the children they did not yearn for in their 20s.) If we give way to what Betty wants *now*, we could well be *preventing* what she will want in the future. *This* is part of the harm that we might be doing. Whereas if we do not accede to her demand now, we leave it open for *her* to decide these matters in the future. In other words, if we are now governed by the principle of non-maleficence, we can thereby allow the principle of autonomy to govern what it should properly govern in the future.

So for these reasons, and given the facts as supposed, it seems to me that Dr H should not accede to Betty's demand for a hysterectomy. This is a case which I think belongs to section N/A of the grid, where non-maleficence overrides autonomy.

In **Case 9**, the doctor has certainly compromised himself, ethically speaking. In telling Mr Y that he was sure that the tablets would help, Dr X has not actually lied. (He *was* sure that the tablets would help, and he was right!) But he has deceived Mr Y. Mr Y asked for sleeping pills, and Dr X responded by giving him tablets which Mr Y believed, and which Dr X *intended* Mr Y to believe, *were* sleeping tablets; whereas in fact they were tablets that had no medical efficacy. Dr X has not been truthful, and in that way he has breached the principle of autonomy. But he has done so for Mr Y's good. For the doctor has correctly recognised that Mr Y's problem was anxiety, and that he could be relieved of his anxiety, and so get good sleep, without sleeping pills (which can have side-effects, and can become addictive, and can be the means of fatal self-harm), so long as Mr Y *believed* that the tablets he was taking were sleeping pills. So Dr X has achieved the good that Mr Y wanted without the harm that sleeping pills might cause – but at the cost of truthfulness. If the deception is justified, this case belongs in section B/A of the grid, where beneficence overrides autonomy. But *is this* a case of justified deception? Truthfulness really matters, and we ought to feel very serious moral qualms about professional deception. We may well believe that honesty is important for its own sake, on deontological grounds. But we can also point out that a professional's honesty is a vital foundation for the patient's or client's *trust*. (We have stressed the importance of this in the previous chapter.) For the professional to be able to serve the client effectively, the client needs to be able to trust the professional; but trust would be *betrayed* by deception, and it would be *destroyed* if the client came to suspect the deception. Thus, deception can destroy the professional-client relationship, and so it can destroy the opportunity for the professional to offer effective service to the client. And in this way deception can violate not only the principle of autonomy, but also the principle of non-maleficence: it can do harm to the relationship upon which effective care depends. On the other hand, there are arguments in favour of Dr X's deception. First, some would feel that the amount of genuine good that Dr X thereby manages to do for Mr Y is sufficient to outweigh the minor deception in which he engages. Secondly, it might be felt that Mr Y's neurotic anxiety impairs his autonomy: it renders him unable properly to appreciate his own condition and what he needs for relief. And so the requirements of the principle of autonomy are here less weighty than those of beneficence. A third and related claim is that Dr X is *not* acting in a way that is *fundamentally* untruthful: he has correctly recognised the truth about Mr Y's condition, and he is acting consistently with that truth by treating the condition in the best way for Mr Y. He is telling Mr Y *the truth* when he tells him that he is sure that the tablets will help; and this is the really important truth in the case. Mr Y's awareness of the exact nature of what is happening would interfere with treatment that is consistent with this truth; whereas if the treatment is successful, then perhaps Dr X will later be able to explain to Mr Y what he has in fact done, helping Mr Y to appreciate that his anxiety had been the problem, and that Dr X was in fact acting for his good – thereby ensuring that the relationship of trust is maintained, or at least restored. We need to be careful, here, that we are not merely inventing cunning rationalisations for our deceptive behaviour. But the argument just mentioned surely does offer a useful test to apply when asking whether deception can be justified. In my treatment which involves this deception, am I trying to help the patient to reach a point where I can fully and openly explain what I have been doing, and where the patient can understand how I have been acting for his good – and where, therefore, the patient can see that, even though I have deceived him, his trust in me has not been misplaced?

In **Case 10**, the doctor is faced with an agonising ethical conflict. He owes the mother the truth – the truth she has expressly requested; the truth about *her* baby; the truth which at that moment is more important to her than any other. But the doctor is also fighting for her life, and he knows that the truth could do her such harm that it may cause her death. The principle of autonomy speaks in favour of telling her the truth. The principle of non-maleficence speaks in favour of withholding the truth from her. If the doctor's overriding duty here is to tell the mother the truth, then the case belongs in section A/N of the grid, where autonomy outweighs non-maleficence. But if his overriding duty is to avoid the harm that the truth would cause, the case belongs in section N/A, where non-maleficence outweighs autonomy. How ought the doctor to decide?

This kind of case has been discussed for centuries, and different commentators have offered different opinions about how it should be dealt with.[6] The case offers an acute instance of a conflict that arises often in medicine and other professions. Professionals often need to deliver bad news – news that can sometimes do crushing harm to the patient or client. Errors can be made at opposite extremes. Sometimes in medicine, the truth is hidden forever from the patient, who is allowed to go on believing that there is a hopeful medical prognosis until he eventually dies in a narcotic-induced unconsciousness. This veil of secrecy and lies is surely wrong – not least because it prevents the patient from taking responsibility for how *he* deals with *his* situation, which is the central concern of the principle of autonomy. But at the other extreme, the truth is sometimes blurted out or delivered with a clinical detachment that is in its effect devoid of compassion, and the patient is devastated by it. There are many cases where the truth does need to be told even though it will do harm – cases that do properly belong in section A/N of the grid. But in these cases, ethically sensitive professionals will do what they can do to mitigate the harm. It may be that the truth can be withheld until the patient is better able to bear it; or that it can be delivered sparingly, over time, in a way that allows the patient to become better able to cope with it. The professional should take pains to ensure that the right sort of support is in place to help the patient to bear and deal with the truth. And the professional should also take pains to ensure that the truth is not delivered in such a way as to cause the patient to give up *realistic* hope. Sometimes, though the situation is grim, there is a genuine chance of a good outcome, but a chance that can be realised only if the patient optimistically fights for that outcome. The professional must deliver the news in such a way as not to cause the patient to abandon this hope.

In Case 10, the doctor knows that, although there is no hope for the baby, there is hope for the mother; but only if she fights to live. He must do what he can to prevent her giving up the hope that will move her to fight. He will certainly want to withhold the truth from her until it is not too terrible for her to bear; until she is strong enough for it not to overwhelm her and cause her to abandon the hope on which her own life depends. But the problem is made particularly grave by the fact that a mere *withholding* of the truth may be insufficient to prevent her from giving up. She wants to know the answer to her question *now*, and the doctor's silence in response may serve only to confirm her worst fears. We might imagine that in order to motivate her to fight on, the doctor needs to say something like this: "Your baby is all right, but now it's vital that you get well so that you can look after him." And if a lie of this kind is necessary to avoid the harm that would be caused by the truth, then the case has become a particularly extreme instance of the problem raised by Case 9 – the problem of whether deception can be justified. (In Case 9, the deception was primarily aimed at good for the patient; it was to help him by relieving his sleeplessness. In Case 10, the primary motivation for deception would be the avoidance of harm – the harm caused by the dreadful truth.) Some of the considerations that we noted concerning Case 9 apply also here in Case 10. It can plausibly be claimed that the mother's autonomy is impaired when she asks her question. Her weakened and desperate condition prevents her from being able to respond to the truth with free and proper judgement. The very fact that the truth might cause her to surrender her life now, but would not cause her to do so if she were well, is enough to show that she cannot function as her own truly autonomous self at the moment, and thus that life is more important than truth in this situation. But it can also be claimed that deception would constitute a frightful betrayal of the mother's trust in the doctor – a betrayal so grave that it could be extremely difficult to restore trust later on. So here again, deception can violate the principle of non-maleficence as well as the principle of autonomy. (And thus the principle of non-maleficence is itself divided in what it says about this case: it speaks against telling the harmful truth, but it also speaks against doing harm to the therapeutic relationship of trust.) In discussing Case 9, we suggested that it can be useful to ask whether, in opting for deception, we are seeking to bring the patient to the point where we can fully explain what we have done and how it was required for the patient's good. And if that is our aim, we might hope that, despite having learned of our deception, the patient's trust in us can be restored. But we need to recognise that the situations in which we explain the truth and seek to restore the relationship of trust would be very different in Cases 9 and 10. The doctor in Case 9, if he discloses his deception at all, will be doing so within the happy situation in which Mr Y is enjoying relief from his sleeplessness. But if the mother in Case 10 survives, she will certainly be aware that deception has occurred. She will be faced with the terrible truth that her baby is dead – and that her doctor *lied* to her about *this*. And as I remarked, she might feel so betrayed by this deception that her trust in the doctor cannot be restored. All the same, there will be no question of future trust if the mother dies. And so the doctor might feel that, in this regard, the problem of how he can restore her trust will be a good problem to have – a problem that will arise only if he can succeed in helping her to survive now.

What should the doctor in Case 10 do? Where is the right balance between autonomy and non-maleficence in this case?

In discussing Cases 4 and 5, we saw how the requirements of justice might outweigh those of autonomy and non-maleficence. And in Case 1, we saw how justice might trump the requirements of beneficence. Case 1 was a case which raised the problem of how a limited resource ought to be distributed over a range of needy patients. It was, in part, what is often called a *micro-allocation* problem: how should this *particular* resource be allocated among these *particular* patients? (How should Dr P distribute her limited time among the patients presented to her – Mrs Q, on the one hand, and the patients in the waiting room, on the other?) But there are also *macro-allocation* problems, where the distribution of the limited resource needs to be determined at a much more general or wide-scale level. How much of the limited public funds ought to be spent on healthcare? How much of the limited public healthcare budget ought to be spent on *this* kind of medical facility (e.g., very expensive, technologically advanced units in large metropolitan hospitals), and how much ought to be spent on *that* kind (e.g., clinics in remote rural areas)? What does *justice* require on these matters, and in what ways should the requirements of justice be tempered by the requirements of the other principles? In **Case 11**, we are presented with a macro-allocation problem – of a rather unusual kind.

It might be argued that justice requires that everyone have equal access to life-saving resources. And a great deal of life-threatening kidney disease occurs because the required resource is not distributed equally: most of us have twice as much of that resource as we really need, while some of us have none of it. (This is not really a case in which the resource is *limited*. There is more than enough of it, but it is unequally distributed.) The proposed system of national service in live kidney donation would ensure that everyone had access to the required resource. It is true that the system would impose a burden upon the donors. But the system would be *fair* insofar as everyone (or every healthy member of the community who would be suitable as a kidney donor) would have an *equal chance* of being selected as a donor. It is also true that the system would *compel* the selected donors to surrender a kidney. But compulsion is often required by justice. We saw how Cases 4 and 5 could entail compulsion. The healthcare budget is funded from taxes that we are compelled to pay. We may be compelled to be vaccinated against certain diseases – for our own good, but *also* for the good of others (for these diseases will be eradicated from the community only if a sufficiently high proportion of the community is vaccinated). We might be conscripted as part of a scheme of national military service, where we are required to risk our own lives for the sake of the protection of the whole community.

Nevertheless, most of us seem to baulk at the proposal that there be a system of national service in live kidney donation. (In discussing this case with many classes, I have yet to find a student who clearly supports the proposal.) Is this just a squeamish lack of public spirit on our part? We are concerned, I think, about two things. First, though most of us could manage with just one kidney, it is better to have two. The removal of a kidney leaves the donor facing a riskier future. And the operation to remove the kidney is, of course, a serious and damaging procedure, recovery from which will be painful and slow. Thus, removal of a kidney certainly does harm to the donor patient, even to healthy donors who have a good prognosis. Secondly, I think we are worried about the extent to which our autonomy would be violated. There are various important respects in which we feel that our bodies are private: it is *up to us* to govern what happens to them. And the compulsory removal of an organ of the body would be felt as a particularly serious invasion of our proper bodily integrity – as an attack upon what *we* properly control as persons. It seems to me, in other words, that we feel that the proposed system of compulsory live kidney donation ought to be rejected and consigned to sections N/J and A/J of the grid, where the requirements of the principles of non-maleficence and autonomy override those of the principle of justice.

Are we right to feel that? And even if we are, what about the less drastic proposal concerning post-mortem donation? Does this proposal fall within the proper limits of the principle of justice – where its requirements are not overridden by those of autonomy or non-maleficence? What do you think?

Case 12 is drawn from my own experience. The university in Johannesburg at which I taught in the 1990s was connected to a number of public hospitals that possessed fine neo-natal intensive care units. But because many more premature babies were born than could be provided with intensive care, the policy of these units was to admit only babies with a birth weight of 1,000 grams or more. This rule was applied, as a matter of fairness, to all babies across all the hospitals. I arrived at one of these hospitals on a Tuesday morning to give an invited lecture on ethics, and before the lecture the consultant in charge took me on a ward round. He showed me this baby, who had been born on the Saturday night, and who had, "by mistake", been admitted to the ICU. The baby was still in the unit, and still doing well. The hospital team had not had the heart to remove the baby from the ICU – and send him to his likely death. Nor did I have the heart to challenge their decision. I gained the impression that no eligible baby had had to be turned away from the ICU since the Saturday night. But no-one could be sure of what demand there would be over the coming days. The ICU team were pressing on in their care for the baby, hoping for the best.

I think that the ICU team were made deeply uneasy by the suggestion that, *having been* caring for the baby since Saturday evening, they could *now* withdraw their care and reject him. And I think that we are right to be troubled by the thought that care, once begun, can be withdrawn. It seems to me that we feel that when a doctor commences treatment, he or she enters into a kind of relationship with the patient: a relationship that involves a *commitment* to care – a commitment that is abandoned if care is withdrawn. And we do not want doctors to be the kind of people who can easily abandon these relationships. We do not want them to be the kind of people who "have the heart" to reject the patients they have been caring for.

Even so, the ICU team were supposed to be operating under a rule that was to be applied fairly to all patients. The 1,000-grams rule had been chosen by the hospital policymakers in order to have a proper way to deal with the painful resource allocation decisions with which they were faced. The rule was the outcome of their attempt to determine a just distribution of their neo-natal ICU resources. They were seeking to apply the principle of justice. (We noted earlier that it can be horrendously difficult to determine what justice *does* require in this kind of situation.) And the hospitals were applying this rule impartially – as justice does require. But this ICU team had breached the rule in order to care for the baby. Would the team have been right to feel that this was a case in which the claims of beneficence trumped those of justice – and so a case which belongs to section B/J of the grid?

We can fairly readily feel that beneficence takes precedence when it is contested by a rule that we do not consider to be what we might call a *fundamental* rule of justice. The doctor in Case 1 was faced with a similar, though much less grave, contest. She might have had a rule by which she limited appointments to, say, 15 minutes; and this rule might have given her a reasonable procedure for balancing the needs of her patients with the need to have some time for each patient, and with the need for her practice to pay its way (not to mention the needs arising from her duties outside her practice – her duties to her family, her duty to preserve her own health and wellbeing, and so on). Justice would then require her to apply this rule in a way that is fair – to apply it impartially, in the same way to all patients. But it is not as if her patients had some fundamental right to 15 minutes of her time, as opposed to 10 minutes, or 20 minutes, or some other figure. And we can easily imagine situations in which it would be right for her to override the demands of this rule for the sake of some more pressing need. (Perhaps Case 1 was not one of those situations. But if Mrs Q had collapsed in the consulting room, it surely would have been right for Doctor P to keep the other patients waiting while attending to this emergency.) Now the 1,000-grams rule in Johannesburg was rather similar to the 15-minute appointment rule – except that it was in effect deciding questions of life or death. It was not as if babies of less than 1,000 grams, on the one hand, and those of a higher birth weight, on the other, had fundamentally different claims upon the hospitals: each surely had a right to the best care that the hospitals could provide. It was not as if the heavier babies deserved that care in a way that the other babies did not. And it was not as if the lower-weight babies would not benefit from the ICU facilities. (Many babies with a birth weight of very much less than 1,000 grams can do very well indeed, so long as they receive proper intensive care; and these are the babies who need those facilities most.) The 1,000-grams rule was what the policymakers felt was their best attempt to find a workable rule that would allow the limited ICU facilities to be used in the most responsible way. They felt, I think, that the application of this rule would save the greatest number of lives over the long run. (But they possessed only slender evidence that this was the right rule to achieve that end. And there was the further question of whether that was the right end to pursue.)

Moreover, it seems to me that there are serious reasons why we do not want doctors and other carers to find it *easy* to ration their limited life-saving resources, and easy, therefore, to withhold care from the patients rejected by the rationing procedure. The ethos of medicine, at its best, consists of a deep commitment to provide care for *whoever* is in need of that care. This commitment does not discriminate between patients. It may need to set priorities according to more or less pressing needs; but it does not regard some needy patients as worthy of care and others as unworthy. In requiring carers to ration their limited resources, we are requiring them to discriminate between the patients who will receive their care and those who won't; we are requiring them to adopt a perspective which runs counter to their proper *unqualified* commitment to care for whoever is in need of their care. Furthermore, we are requiring the carers *to decide who shall live and who shall die.*[7] And this decision, we may well feel, is not a decision that any one of us has the right to make. We are mere mortals, extending care to other mere mortals in need. What entitles *us* to determine which of these needy mortals shall live and which shall die? We may well feel that anyone who can readily make such decisions is the kind of person who belongs nowhere near the caring professions.

And yet rationing decisions need to be made, and there need to be people who are prepared to accept the responsibility to make those decisions in the wisest and most sensitive way possible. And the rationing principles, whatever they are, ought to be applied *fairly*. The family of a baby rejected under the 1,000-grams rule may well feel that a wrong decision was made in Case 12. Did we do the wrong thing in that case?[8]

There are many other possible cases we could consider; but our review of the cases above shows how there could be a kind of case for each of the sections of the grid, for we have imagined at least one possible case for each section. And this confirms the view of Beauchamp and Childress that each of the four principles is a *prima facie* principle: it can both override and be overridden by any of the other principles. The cases we have discussed above may be difficult to resolve, but many of them are relatively *neat* cases, in that they involve some clash between merely two of the principles. Some of them were not quite so neat as that: Cases 4, 5 and 11, for instance, involved a tension between one principle and *two* of the others – a tension between the principle of justice, on the one hand, and the principles of autonomy and non-maleficence, on the other. And many of the ethical problems we face in professional life are not so neat: they may arise from situations in which perhaps all four of the principles make relevant claims. But in these more complex situations, our task will still be the same: we will need to find the right balance between the claims of the different principles.

I have pointed out that workers within the wider caring professions might face any one of the kinds of healthcare cases we have considered above. And of course, they will face cases of many further kinds, some of which will have no particular connection to healthcare. Some of these cases will involve more than two relevant principles. And some will, in another way, be more complex and less neat than those we have considered above: they will be cases in which a number of different *persons* are involved, and it will be much harder to draw a neat distinction between the professional's client, on the one hand, and third parties who are not clients, on the other. Think, for instance, of a typical social work case:

> A single mother is living with her three children in public housing. The family has been receiving support for some time, but their situation has continued to deteriorate. The mother is heavily affected by alcohol and drugs. She wishes to care for her children, all of whom are under the age of ten, but the care she in fact provides is very poor and the conditions of the home are dangerously squalid. The children wish to remain with their mother, but their health, their education, and their general welfare are being seriously undermined in their current conditions.

The social workers who have responsibility for this case will, of course, wish to treat the case as that of a *whole family*. But the interests of the individuals within the family could diverge from one another. What is best for the children may well be different, at least in the short term, from what is best for the mother. The social workers may need to regard *each* member of the family as an individual client to whom they have a duty of care – a duty to act in a way that is properly governed by the four principles. And they will need to do their best to discharge this duty while keeping properly in view the interests of the family as a whole. Clearly, then, this is a situation in which there is a *complex* of clients – though a complex within which the four principles can still be applied to each member of the complex in turn.

Even so, if the situation is one in which one or other person is the *primary* client, it can help to see how the relevant principles apply to the case if that person is thought of as the one to whom the principles of beneficence, non-maleficence and autonomy apply, and the other involved persons are thought of as those whose interests are considered under the principle of justice. Because the principle of justice requires us to consider *all* the interests of affected third parties, this way of thinking about the case should offer no improper advantage to the interests of the primary client. But it can make our thinking about the case somewhat less messy than if we have to apply each of the four principles in turn to every one of the persons involved in the case. (The possible messiness can be seen in the following way. Imagine, for instance, that there are four persons who are fairly directly involved in a case. If the professional with a duty of care is thinking about what each principle requires in relation to each of those persons, she will need to consider what justice requires in relation to each of those persons. But the requirements of justice will overlap with each other; for the persons other than person 1 overlap with the persons other than person 2, and so on. And the requirements of justice will overlap with the requirements of the other principles; for the requirements of justice in relation to person 1 will overlap with the requirements of beneficence in relation to person 2, and so on. It might be thought, then, that we can dispense with the principle of justice in such a case, and simply consider what the other three principles require concerning each of the four persons, given that those three principles embrace all the interests of each of those persons. But this would be a mistake, for justice requires that we consider not merely the interests of the other persons within that group of four, but also those of anyone else outside that group who is affected by what happens in the case. Thus, we need to keep the principle of justice in the picture. And so it will help to keep our thinking about the case somewhat more clearly organised if we can properly regard *one* of those four persons as the primary client, and everyone else who is involved or who could be affected as a party whose interests are protected by the principle of justice. But this neat way of organising our thinking won't always be possible; and where it is not possible, we must simply keep a careful, clear perspective on the application of the principles in relation to everyone concerned.)

Let us round off our discussion of the four principles by considering how they apply to two more fairly typical social work cases that have no very direct connection to healthcare. I invite you to think about each case and consider what the social worker ought to do before you read my review of the case. You are once again identifying the principles that apply to the case, and working out the right balance between the claims of the principles.[9]

Case 13

An elderly couple are referred by their next-door neighbour to the Aged Care Assessment team. The neighbour is concerned that the couple, who live with their adult daughter and her husband, are rarely seen and that screams can be heard from the house.

When the social worker visits the house, she finds a frail elderly couple who admit that financial and physical abuse is occurring. The daughter gets frustrated with the father in particular. She has pushed him off his chair, locked him in the bathroom, and hit him with a broom in frustration at his physical frailty. In addition, the daughter collects all her parents' pension money, providing board and lodging in return. The daughter's husband has recently been retrenched, and they depend on their income from the couple just to pay the grocery bill each fortnight.

Despite having lost control over their money, and despite living with a potentially violent carer, who is clearly under considerable stress herself, the couple refuse to take any action against their daughter. They argue in her defence and say that although they acknowledge that there have been difficulties, they would rather stay with their own family than go to a strange place where they are not known.

The social worker persuades them to consider accepting some personal care through the Home Care Service in order to take the strain from the daughter. Although their decision to stay in the situation is not the decision she would have made, the social worker decides to respect the wishes of this couple, who are both cognitively competent. When she approaches the daughter about arranging some home care assistance for her parents, the daughter reluctantly agrees to a trial period, "providing it doesn't cost too much".

Case 14

Phillip is a social worker in a mental health team. He has a 25-year-old client, Peter, who has been given various diagnoses over the years. Peter's symptoms subside when he takes his medication; but he does not like taking medication and will do so only under supervision. When not on medication, Peter has been violent, particularly towards his mother and sisters. Peter currently lives in a boarding house. The community nurse usually visits him each day to supervise his medication. For the last few days, however, Peter has not been at home at the boarding house when the nurse has called. He has been receiving counselling from Phillip for about three months, and Phillip is requested to find out what has happened to Peter. Peter does not want his family to know his whereabouts and has specifically requested that they not be informed of his progress or any other details of his life.

When Phillip visits the boarding house, Peter is still not there and has not been seen for a week. The manager is pleased to see Phillip and volunteers much information about Peter's behaviour at the boarding house. "Usually a quiet bloke," is the manager's perception, but he reports that lately Peter has been even more withdrawn and has been seen dressing strangely and muttering to himself. The manager wants to know "what's been going on with the team" to allow Peter to get into this state. He also asks what sort of medication Peter is taking, how long he has been ill and for other details of Peter's life and condition. Phillip feels very awkward about answering these questions, but the manager is persistent. "After all," says the manager, "I have to deal with day-to-day life around here and it's very hard if I don't know the facts."

When Phillip returns to the office, there is a telephone message from Peter's mother, Beverley. She rings again while Phillip is there and he takes the call. Beverley sounds very distressed. "Some friends of my eldest daughter said they saw Peter hanging around the railway station dressed in army fatigues and carrying a knife in his belt," she says. "Please tell me what is happening. He has been violent before. My husband is away and when Peter gets in one of his moods, there's no knowing what he'll do. What have you been talking to him about? I thought he was supposed to be supervised with his medication since your team became involved. But no one tells the relatives anything. Then they cop it when things go wrong. You people come and go and can leave your jobs at any time. Peter is our boy and we always end up carrying the can no matter what all you professionals think. Please tell me what is happening. I am worried for the safety of my family."

In the interests of the family, Phillip decides to break his promise to Peter that he would not tell his family about his situation. He describes his worries that Peter is off his medication and repeats what the manager has told him.

"Please try to find him," Beverley pleads. "I'm so glad you told me. I think I'll get my brother over just in case. I'll ring you if he turns up here. He usually does sooner or later, once he goes off his tablets. Is your after-hours number still the same?"

Presuming, now, that you have thought about the cases yourself, let us review each one. Once again, I shall not try to provide a full resolution of these cases; I shall simply make some fairly brief observations about the applications of the four principles, to provide a basis for you to think about the cases more thoroughly.

The social worker in **Case 13** can regard the elderly couple as her clients, and she is rightly concerned for their welfare – with what would be for their good. She feels that it would be best for them to be removed from an abusive situation. But what is suggested by beneficence is here in tension with autonomy, for the elderly couple wish to remain where they are. The social worker feels that this is a case in which autonomy represents the overriding requirement. But she is also taking some measures to provide help for the couple and to lessen the danger to them. Beneficence is still playing a role, though in a way that is subordinate to autonomy. The social worker is no doubt sensitive also to the possible relevance of the principles of non-maleficence and justice. She does not want to intervene in a way that could cause more harm than good (by removing the couple from a place of familiarity and support, for example; or by adding destructive tension to an important but already strained relationship with the daughter). And she has an eye on the needs of the affected third parties, the daughter and her husband (while also being aware that there could be a case for decisive action *against* the daughter).

Is the social worker finding the right balance between these various considerations? Is she right to feel that she should support the couple in their wish to remain where they are? (She has noted that their autonomy is not impaired by mental incompetence. But could they be stating their wish under duress, or because they feel under pressure from their daughter? Should the social worker be doing more in order to eliminate this possibility?) Or are the danger to and the abuse of the couple so serious that the social worker ought not to accede to their wish to stay where they are? If that is so, what steps can she properly take? On the other hand, if she is right to accede to their wish, is there more that she should be doing in order to advance their welfare and to protect them from abuse? How should her course of action be determined?

In **Case 14**, Peter is Phillip's client, and Phillip is rightly concerned to protect Peter's interests. But he also needs to be very concerned to protect the interests of possibly endangered third parties, including the members of Peter's family. The principle of justice requires that urgent steps be taken to find Peter and get him back onto his medication. And the requirements of the principle of beneficence would seem here to coincide with those of justice, for it will be better for Peter to be back on his medication, and it will be better for him – as well as for endangered third parties – if he poses no danger to others. (We shudder to imagine what could happen if the situation were to escalate and Peter became involved in a stand-off with the police.)

There is a tension, however, between those principles, on the one hand, and the principle of autonomy, on the other. Peter is unlikely to want to take his medication. Given that his autonomy is presumably impaired in his current condition, and given the need to protect others, his wish not to take his medication can scarcely be overriding. The more interesting aspect of the tension concerns what Phillip is saying to the manager of the boarding house and to Peter's family. Phillip is breaching confidentiality, and he is doing so having promised Peter that he would not provide those details to the family. Promise-keeping is a particularly important kind of truthfulness. When we make a promise to someone, we provide a guarantee of what we will do – a guarantee that entitles that person to act on the basis of that guarantee. So promise-breaking is, *in effect*, the final stage in a process of deception: it renders our guarantee *false*. And thus, like other kinds of deception, it involves a serious breach of trust. We have considered the permissibility of deception and of betrayals of trust in discussing some of the earlier cases. What can usefully be carried over from those discussions to this case? Ought Phillip to have given his promise to Peter in the first place? Perhaps Phillip had good reason to believe that Peter would not accept his services as a social worker unless he, Phillip, promised not to provide information to the family. If that were so, would it make a difference to whether Phillip ought to have made the promise? And whether or not Phillip ought to have made the promise in the first place, ought he to be bound by it now? How much weight ought he attach to the fact that if he talks to Peter's family and the boarding house manager, then his caring relationship with Peter – and therefore his care for Peter – is likely to be seriously harmed by his breaches of confidentiality? (What further weight, in other words, does the principle of non-maleficence add to the principle of autonomy's support for maintaining confidentiality?) But in any case, are these considerations outweighed by the need to breach confidentiality? Anyone who needs to be acting in a way that is important for Peter's good needs to know enough about Peter's situation to be able to judge *how* to act for his good. Even the boarding house manager will need to have *some* relevant information if he is to play a reliable role within Peter's care environment. So the principle of beneficence speaks in favour of the provision of *appropriate* information to those whose actions will affect Peter. (But is Phillip providing only appropriate information?) However, as we noted at the outset, the urgent need at the moment arises from the requirements of the principle of justice. The people who may be endangered by Peter have a right to be protected from that danger, and they have a right to know what they would need to know in order to take proper steps to protect themselves.

What is the right balance between these various considerations? What course of action, on Phillip's part, will strike that proper balance?

Conclusion

Our discussion of all these different cases has illustrated my earlier point that the four principles are *limited* in what they can do for us. There are situations in which it is very difficult to know what a particular principle (e.g., the principle of justice) would entail in that situation. There are many situations in which it is difficult to know how the right balance is to be struck between the different applicable principles. There are moral aspects of some situations that are not illuminated by the four principles at all. And even where we can see that a principle does apply to a situation, we still need to work out the specific practical form that this application should take. For all these reasons, the four principles do not provide us with a *formula* for ethically correct action. Nevertheless, our discussion has also shown how the principles are *useful*. We noted earlier that there are many situations in which our ethical duties are quite straightforward, and the principles can help us to see these duties clearly. And our discussion of the hard cases has shown us that even in the situations in which there is some ethical tension and confusion, the four principles provide a *helpful framework* for the assessment of the situation. By applying each principle, we can illuminate the moral aspects of the situation. We can see what is at stake. And the more we bring each ethical aspect into clear light, the more we shall be able to recognise what is of overriding importance.

And we can consciously employ the four principles as guidelines in our professional practice. We shall be doing well if we are constantly asking ourselves: "How can I act for the good here? How do I need to avoid harm? In what ways should I be ensuring that I am respecting the patient or client's autonomy? In what ways should I be concerned about the need to act justly? And how do these various concerns weigh against each other?" Each of us should be conscientiously asking these questions, and conscientiously *practising* the conduct indicated by their answers. Our doing this plays an important part in our working towards becoming the kind of persons who can be relied upon to act wisely and well.

Notes

1 Tom L. Beauchamp and James F. Childress, *Principles of Biomedical Ethics*, Eighth Edition (Oxford University Press, Oxford and New York, 2019).

2 Some depth of philosophical foundation for these principles was provided by the English philosopher G. J. Warnock in his important book *The Object of Morality* (Methuen & Co. Ltd., London, 1971).

3 This case and Case 8 are adapted from "Does Doctor Know Best?", Programme No. 2 in the series *Ethics in America*, produced by Columbia University Seminars on Media and Society, 1989, and distributed as a video instructional series by Annenberg Learner. This excellent programme displays a panel of experts in their ethical exploration of a hypothetical case.

4 See note 3.

5 G. R. McLean, "H.I.V. Infection and a Limit to Confidentiality", in *South African Journal on Human Rights*, Vol. 12, Part 3, 1996, pp. 452–66.

6 Helmut Thielicke mentions the case, and reports various commentators' pronouncements upon it, in the course of a fascinating general discussion of situations in which we might be unable to avoid moral compromises concerning truth-telling, and of what such situations indicate about our own moral condition and the moral condition of the world in which we must operate: Helmut Thielicke, *Theological Ethics*, Volume I: *Foundations* (A. & C. Black, London, 1968), Chapter 27.

7 *The Doctor as Judge of Who Shall Live and Who Shall Die* is the title of a booklet by Helmut Thielicke. See also note 8.

8 It might well be thought that *any* decision in Case 12 would be wrong – or at least deeply morally questionable. Like Case 10, and perhaps some of the other cases we have considered, Case 12 involves not just a clash but a profound tension between different moral principles. We may well feel, therefore, that we are fooling ourselves if we think that there is a *satisfactory* resolution of such cases. We may feel that any decision we make in such a case is deeply unsatisfactory, *and* that it is a deeply unsatisfactory fact that *we cannot avoid* making a decision (for even the choice to do nothing is in effect a decision in a quite particular direction). The very situation in which we face such a decision is, we may feel, a deeply morally unsatisfactory state of affairs, from which we cannot escape. If we do feel these things, then we have some sense of part of what Helmut Thielicke is referring to as "metaphysical guilt", which he believes ought to accompany even our best decisions in such cases: Helmut Thielicke, *The Doctor as Judge of Who Shall Live and Who Shall Die* (Fortress Press, Philadelphia, 1976).

9 Cases 13 and 14 have been formulated and used during recent years by Charles Sturt University teachers in the ethics of social work. Case 13 was contributed to this teaching programme by R. Bunt.

Part B
Applications

6
Euthanasia

In this second part of the book, I want to discuss a couple of particular but very substantial ethical problems. I am going to use these problems as case studies for the application of some of the basic equipment that we have gathered in the first part of the book. As we tackle these problems, I want us to see what mileage we can extract from our commonly accepted moral principles – particularly the four-principles framework. But I want us also to note places where the different philosophical theories, and different world-view commitments, will inevitably influence the views of those who take part in the discussion of these problems. In this chapter, we shall consider the first of these problems – euthanasia.

Is euthanasia permissible? This is a very topical question: it is currently being discussed in many parts of the world. It presents a complicated problem – or rather, a cluster of connected but distinct problems. There is first the basic problem of whether some particular act of euthanasia could be morally permissible. This is itself a complicated problem. But beyond it is the further problem of the *general* attitude towards euthanasia that ought to be taken by professional ethics. This is a distinct problem because it could perhaps turn out to be true, for instance, that although some particular *act* of euthanasia could be permissible, it would be ethically irresponsible of the caring professions to accept as a general principle that euthanasia is a legitimate option within medical practice. And then there is the yet further problem of the attitude that ought to be taken by the *law*.

In this chapter, I shall try to present what I hope is a helpful overview of some of the main aspects of this complicated problem. And I shall suggest a way of thinking about it which is not original, but which I hope allows us to find a reasonably clear path towards a resolution of the central problem for *professional ethics*. This suggested resolution will also have implications for the law, but that will not be my main concern. I want us to concentrate upon doing what we

DOI: 10.4324/9781003176541-8

can to assist members of the caring professions to deal with the ethical problem with which they are presented here.[1]

To start with, we need to get some terminology clear and to draw some distinctions. The word "euthanasia" comes from the Greek, where it means simply "a good death" or "dying well". But, as was stressed by the English philosopher Philippa Foot in her landmark article on the subject, we should really use the term only in a much more precise sense – namely, to refer to situations in which death is sought *for the sake of the person who dies*.[2] Thus, even when a patient is provided with a gentle or easy death, it would not be right to describe this death as *euthanasia* when it is brought about not because it is thought to be in *the patient's* interest that he dies, but because, for example, his continued living would place a great burden – of work or of suffering or of cost – upon his family, or a burden of cost upon the medical services provided by society, or for some similar reason involving the interests of others. And by defining "euthanasia" in this proper, precise sense, we can identify certain historic uses of the word as merely outrageous abuses of the term. As we noted in Chapter Three, the Nazi regime had a so-called euthanasia programme under which hundreds of thousands of medically unfit persons, unable to be rehabilitated for work, were exterminated. (This programme became a prototype for the later, much more widespread system of mass murder in the concentration camps.) The fact is, of course, that what was done to those killed under this programme had no connection whatsoever with what was in *their* interests. Here the term "euthanasia" was simply a euphemism for the massacre of persons regarded as undesirable by others in power.

I should point out, however, that in defining the term "euthanasia" in this correct, precise sense, to refer to cases in which the death is sought for the sake of the person who dies, we have not yet said anything about the *morality* of euthanasia. That question still lies before us. For all that the definition shows, it may or may not be morally permissible to seek a person's death intending that death to be for his sake.

We now need to get a quick and rough idea of some distinctions. There is, first, the distinction between active and passive euthanasia. Active euthanasia is the intentional *killing* of a person (for his sake). Passive euthanasia is the intentional *allowing of a person to die* (for his sake). Secondly, there is a three-part distinction between voluntary, involuntary and non-voluntary euthanasia. Voluntary euthanasia (whether active or passive) is euthanasia *at the express request of the person who dies*. Involuntary euthanasia is *contrary to the expressed wish of the person who dies* – that is, he wishes to go on living. And non-voluntary euthanasia occurs *without the express request of the person who dies*, either because he is not asked what he wishes or because he is unable to give an answer to this question – perhaps because he is comatose, or infantile, or senile, or in some other way incompetent to state a wish. Again, in defining these terms, we have not yet said anything about the morality of what is being referred to. (You might think that involuntary euthanasia is defined in such a way that it is *obviously* immoral: how could it ever be permissible to kill a patient against his will? But it is possible to *argue* that there could be cases in which a patient *wants* to go on living even though it would be *best for him* if he died; and that in such cases there is a very real moral question of what we ought to do. So, for the time being, let us simply note the issue.)

And finally, we need to define "physician-assisted suicide". This term applies to cases where a person brings about his own death, but with the assistance provided by a doctor – for example, by using lethal drugs supplied by the doctor. Where it is used in contrast to physician-assisted suicide, the term "euthanasia" applies to cases where the death is brought about not by what the patient does to himself, but as a result of the course of action taken by the doctor or some other person – whether that course of action be an act of direct killing (active euthanasia) or a withholding of something that would sustain the patient's life (passive euthanasia).

Now we are ready to do some moral thinking about what we have defined. But I want to begin this by pointing out that the thinking of the caring professions on these issues does not take place within a vacuum: we do not start out with a morally neutral attitude to life, and to the saving or taking of life. We start, rather, with a *presumption*, which is so obvious, and so fundamental to the caring professions, that it is a platitude. Yet it is so important that it is worth stating. This is the presumption that life is a good, and that our duty of care to our patients or clients standardly requires us to sustain and to protect their lives. It is presumed, in other words, that our duty of beneficence entails the sustaining of life, and that our duty of non-maleficence entails our refraining from acting against life. Moreover, it is presumed that we owe the *same* duty of care to *each* of our patients. Our care, in other words, is not to be compromised by judgements about the relative values of our patients' lives. Indeed, our obligation to care, and in particular our obligation to sustain life, is *especially* an obligation to care for *sub-optimal* human life – life which is damaged, or diseased, or deranged, or weak, or helpless.

This presumption that we have a duty to sustain life is so important, and so central to the ethos to which those in the caring professions have committed themselves, that it can hardly be overstated. Nevertheless, powerful as it is, it is a presumption, not an absolute principle. It has its limits. For we are all mortal: our death is an inevitability which medicine cannot finally ward off. And though medicine may have at its disposal the means of prolonging life at a certain level, there are situations in which it can recognise that it ought no longer to employ those means. There are situations in which it ought to desist from further attempts to sustain life, because such attempts would now be out of place.

Some of these limits to the duty to sustain life are relatively clear and uncontroversial; but I think that it will be helpful to spend a little while in considering them, for otherwise they can enter the discussion of euthanasia in a confusing way. Cases in which doctors recognise the proper limits to the duty to sustain life can *look* like cases of euthanasia; but they are different, and need to be distinguished from what is really at issue in the question of euthanasia.[3]

One limit to the duty to sustain life occurs at the point at which life can be sustained only at a vegetative level. The treatment which sustains life only at this level is often called "futile treatment". There could be much discussion of this notion of futile treatment, but I find helpful the account offered by the New Zealand neurosurgeon and bioethicist Grant Gillett.[4] He argues that healthcare professionals have a duty to do all in their power to ensure that their patients can enjoy what he calls an acceptable minimum of human function – that is, a level of function in which things can *matter* to the patient, at least in a primitive personal way. But there are conditions – the genuinely, or irreversibly, persistent vegetative state would be one of these – in which nothing can be done to restore the patient to that level of function: nothing can be done to restore the patient to a point where he can experience or be aware of anything; where he can appreciate in any way the care of others. Yet we may have means that enable us to sustain such a patient's life at this merely vegetative level. Gillett would describe these means as futile: he defines "futile treatment" as treatment which cannot restore the patient to an acceptable minimum of human function. And he argues that we have no duty to sustain life if it can only ever be sustained by futile treatment. For to sustain life in this way is to do nothing from which the patient, as a person, can benefit; it does nothing to serve the patient. It merely prolongs his dying. We might say of these cases, then, that the artificial sustaining of biological life is not the preservation of worthwhile or potentially worthwhile personal life, or the genuine care of a patient, but merely an attempt to deny the mortal human condition.

Another limit to our duty to sustain life occurs at the point where the treatment required to sustain life would impose upon the patient a burden of harm or suffering which is out of all proportion to any good that it can provide. For instance, we may be in a situation in which we can win for our patient a short prolonging of conscious life, but only at the cost – I mean a cost in terms of harm and suffering – of a highly distressing resuscitation, whose outcome is dubious; or of a massive surgical operation, with all its trauma and after-effects. And in such a situation, it may well be judged that the benefit, *for the patient*, simply does not justify the cost, *for the patient*.

Some such decisions will be relatively easy; others will be harder. But it seems to me that the principle of respect for autonomy has an especially important role in such cases: the patient's own wishes are especially significant. Those wishes are always significant, but in these cases it may be that we simply cannot quantify the harm/benefit ratio of the treatment options with which we are presented unless we do so by reference to the patient's own assessment of the matter. For instance, imagine the following situation. Mrs. A, who is 87 years old, is now facing the choice between, on the one hand, another very burdensome surgical operation, which offers the promise of some months of further life of suffering and disability; and, on the other hand, swift death. She prefers not to have the operation. "I feel that my time has come," is the way that she puts it. "I've had a good innings, and I'm ready to be taken by God. And I want to go peacefully with my family around me." Mrs. B, however, who is the same age, in the same condition and facing the same choice, desperately wants to have the operation: her criminal son is due to be released from prison in two months, and it is very important to her that she be reconciled to him before she dies. There we can see, I think, that Mrs. A and Mrs. B are both making perfectly legitimate decisions – *different* decisions, even though their clinical condition is exactly the same. The individual patient's particular weighting of relevant factors may in this kind of way be an essential determinant of the harm/benefit ratio of treatment.

In cases in which life-sustaining treatment exceeds these limits – where it is futile or too burdensome – the standardly presumed connection between our duty of care towards the patient and the sustaining of the patient's life is a connection which comes apart. Where the treatment is futile, it cannot achieve any *good* for the patient; hence it is not required by the duty of beneficence. Where the treatment is too burdensome, the good it would or may achieve is outweighed by the *harm* that it would impose; thus it is contrary to the duty of non-maleficence. Hence we are not obliged to administer treatments of either of these kinds, and may indeed be obliged to withhold or withdraw them.

Now of course, in withholding or withdrawing life-sustaining treatment, we are thereby allowing the patient to die. So it can be argued that, in justifying such a course of action, we have justified cases of passive euthanasia – cases in which, for the patient's sake, we allow him to die, even though we *could* (by administering the futile or unduly burdensome treatment) keep him alive. Nevertheless, I do not think that it is helpful to think of these kinds of case as cases of euthanasia. I do not think that it is splitting hairs to say that what is going on in these kinds of case is *not* that we are *aiming at death*; rather, it is that we are recognising that certain kinds of *treatment* would be out of place. We are recognising that those kinds of treatment are not required by, and may be inconsistent with, our duty of care. But this does not mean that simply by withholding or withdrawing those kinds of treatment, we have fully discharged our duty of care. Our duty of care may still entail many responsibilities even when we can no longer properly sustain life; indeed, that duty may become most acute precisely at this point. I shall have a good deal more to say about this later on. The purpose of the healthcare professional's work is beautifully expressed by the oft-quoted aphorism: "To cure sometimes, to relieve often, to care always."[5] The "always" reminds us that care is essential *not least* when the patient is dying.

There is another traditional doctrine which is worth mentioning here. In discussion of the question of whether doctors ought to press on with treatment to sustain life, a distinction has often been drawn between *ordinary* and *extraordinary* means of treatment. And it has been held that doctors are obliged to persist in ordinary means of treatment; whereas extraordinary means of treatment are not obligatory, but merely optional. Philosophers are typically, and understandably, unimpressed by this doctrine. How, exactly, is extraordinary treatment to be distinguished from ordinary treatment? And even if it can be distinguished, why should the distinction carry any moral weight? Why should the one means of sustaining life be any less, or more, obligatory than the other? These are good questions. But I think that those who have traditionally appealed to this doctrine are driving at something which matters, and which is much better expressed along the lines of what we have just been noting while considering treatment which is futile or too burdensome. What matters is not whether the means of treatment are ordinary or extraordinary – however that is to be determined – but rather the proportionality or otherwise of what the doctors have to do in relation to what they are seeking to achieve. What matters is how the treatment rates against a criterion which we might state roughly as follows: whereas we are normally obliged to pursue the good of the patient (and in the cases we are concerned with here, the good in question is the patient's *life*), we may cease to pursue this good if its attainment would be disproportionately improbable (as when the life-sustaining treatment would be futile) or if its pursuit would be disproportionately harmful (as when the life-sustaining treatment would be too burdensome).

Alongside those limits to the duty to sustain life, there is another kind of case which can look almost indistinguishable from a case of euthanasia, but which arguably belongs to a quite different category. I refer to the sort of procedure which traditionally has been justified by appeal to the *doctrine of double effect*.

This doctrine applies to a kind of action which has two effects: a good effect and a bad effect. According to the doctrine, if you were to perform such an action *intending* to bring about the bad effect, then you would be acting wrongly. But you could perform that same action in a morally acceptable way if your doing so fulfils a number of conditions, which we can state roughly as follows. First, even though you can *foresee* the bad effect of your action, it must be the case that you are not *intending* it, but intending only the good effect. Secondly, the bad effect must be what we might call a side-effect of the action – that is, it must be the case that you are not achieving the good effect *by means of* the bad effect. And thirdly, the good, or the importance, of the good effect must sufficiently outweigh the bad of the bad effect – or, as it is sometimes put, there must be sufficient reason to permit the bad effect. Now, what has all this got to do with our discussion? In the treatment of terminal illness, when palliative care is the only medical option still open and when the relief of pain and discomfort is of major importance, it has commonly been supposed that in certain cases, the dosage of drugs required to provide effective relief may increase to the point where it becomes life-threatening. This may or may not be a real problem in contemporary clinical practice; but let us imagine that it is, for the purpose of the discussion. It means, of course, that the doctor has to choose between, on the one hand, refraining from giving effective relief to a patient who may be suffering terribly, and, on the other hand, giving effective relief which also does, or may, shorten the patient's life. Many doctors, faced with that choice, feel that they are justified in administering the life-shortening dosage of drugs, *even though* they *also* feel that they would *not* be justified in administering that or some other dosage of drugs *in order to kill the patient*. In other words, they feel that there is a real moral difference between giving relief in this way, on the one hand, and directly killing the patient, on the other. They are prepared to do the former, but not the latter. And when this very common view has been challenged, the doctrine of double effect has often been invoked. The dosage of drugs we are talking about has, or may have, two effects – the bad effect of earlier death in addition to the good effect of relief. And it can be argued that the doctrine shows why, whereas it would not be right to act *intending* the bad effect of the patient's death, it can be permissible to give the life-shortening dosage of drugs, because doing so can fulfil the three conditions. First, one is *intending* only the relief, not the shortening of life. Secondly, the relief is not achieved by means of the shortening of life. And thirdly, in the kind of situation we are thinking of, in which the patient is suffering terribly and will die soon anyway, the relief is of tremendous importance, and it does outweigh the significance of a slightly earlier death.

Now we could spend many hours debating the correctness or otherwise of the doctrine of double effect. It is highly controversial in philosophical circles. We can readily note various points at which it can be challenged, from one side or another. Does the doctrine really make sense? Can we *really* claim that someone is not *intending* the bad effect, when he can perfectly clearly see that it will be an effect of the action which he is fully *intentionally* performing? And even if it is true that he is not intending, but merely foreseeing, the bad effect, how is this of any moral importance? We are morally responsible for the foreseeable consequences of our actions (and, indeed, for those consequences of our actions that we *ought* to have foreseen), so the action with that foreseeable consequence must be in the same moral bag as an action with that *intended* consequence. So isn't the doctrine merely a sophistical device for allowing us to deceive ourselves that there is a moral difference between what we are prepared to do and killing – a device that allows us to pretend that we are keeping our hands clean? Moreover, isn't the doctrine perfectly ripe for abuse? Doesn't it offer the ideal smokescreen for the murdering doctor who despatches his terminally ill patients with large doses of morphine? For he can always claim that he didn't *intend* the death of his patient, but only relief from pain and distress.

You will perhaps be relieved to hear that I do not have the space in this chapter to review that long debate. Philosophically problematic as the doctrine is, and ripe for abuse as it most certainly is, I do think that it is gesturing at something important. And I share the traditional view that there is a morally important distinction to be drawn between giving the kind of life-shortening dosage of drugs that we have been thinking about, on the one hand, and directly killing the patient, on the other. The doctor who will do the former but not the latter would certainly choose a less dangerous means of providing effective relief *if one were available*. And this shows that his *aim*, his *purpose*, is not the death but the relief of the patient. In that sense, we can argue that the relief but not the death is what he intends. All the same, he must of course shoulder responsibility for what he is foreseeably bringing about; and he can do so with moral propriety *only* if the relief at which he is aiming is important and great enough to render morally tolerable the shortening of life. In other words, what would otherwise be an unjustified breach of the duty of non-maleficence is tolerable only because of the strength of the demands of the duty of beneficence. Once again, we can put this last point in terms of the proportionality or otherwise of what we have to do in relation to what we are aiming to bring about, along the lines of the following rough criterion: whereas we are normally obliged to avoid harm to the patient (and in the cases we are concerned with here, the harm in question is the patient's earlier death), we may pursue the good (relief from pain and distress) at the risk of this harm if the good is important and probable enough to outweigh the harm (quantified as a function of its risk).[6]

The various kinds of case that we have so far discussed – cases of withholding or withdrawing life-sustaining treatment which is futile or unduly burdensome, and cases of administering pain-relieving drugs which will, or may, shorten the patient's life – are relatively uncontroversial. And my treatment of them has, I think, been consistent with a traditional medical ethical outlook. But I have taken some pains over these cases because I want us to be able to draw some real distinctions between them and cases of euthanasia. For it might be argued that each of these cases involves a course of action which is morally indistinguishable from euthanasia; and hence, that if we accept those courses of action as permissible, then consistency demands that we should also accept euthanasia as permissible. In each of these courses of action (the withholding of life-sustaining treatment, the administering of life-shortening drugs), the known (or at least probable) consequence of the action is the death of the patient. But this is exactly the same consequence as the consequence of the course of action that we describe as euthanasia. So these various courses of action, including euthanasia, are all morally on a par. If we accept some, we ought to accept them all.

But I reject that line of argument. It is the kind of argument which would be appealing to the consequentialist. But I have rejected consequentialism. The consequences of our actions are not the only things that matter, morally speaking. Our intentions and purposes matter. And if some kinds of action are intrinsically right, or wrong, then it matters whether I am intending to perform an action of such a kind. As I have tried to indicate, the intentions and purposes involved in the courses of action we have so far accepted can be distinguished – importantly distinguished – from those involved in euthanasia. In a case of what is properly called euthanasia, the end or object one is aiming at is the patient's death; one acts with the intention and purpose of bringing about the patient's death. By contrast, in the kinds of case we have discussed, one is not acting in order to bring about the patient's death. As the English ethicist David Atkinson puts it, these courses of action involve choices for life rather than choices for death: "They seek to enable a person to live as fully as possible even while dying."[7]

Still, though the courses of action we have so far discussed are to be distinguished from what is properly called euthanasia, this does not show us what we ought to say about euthanasia. We have not yet seen whether or not euthanasia is morally permissible – and here, at last, we come to our central issue. Let us launch into it by considering what we may regard as a *paradigm case of euthanasia*. This will be a case which unambiguously involves an intention to kill, and a course of action which directly brings about that end – such as the administering of a lethal injection. And the argument for such a course of action surely has its best chance of success when it concerns a situation in which the patient has expressly requested this act of euthanasia. So we are considering, as our paradigm case, voluntary active euthanasia. I think that what we say about this case will enable us also to evaluate the other cases of euthanasia.

So, what ought we to say about this case? The question we are now asking finds itself located in the neighbourhood of weighty and fundamental philosophical issues. There is the issue of the ethics of killing – whether it can ever be right, and if it can, under precisely what conditions. There are also metaphysical issues, or issues concerning what we might refer to as the significance or meaning of life and death. For instance, let's recall the different world-view commitments we compared in Chapter Three, and consider how they would variously colour one's thinking about voluntary euthanasia. The atheistic world-view commitment might express itself here in the following kind of way: "My life is my own; I am my own master, subject to no other authority. And this life, with its suffering or happiness, is the only life there is." Whereas the theistic world-view commitment might be expressed here as follows: "My life is a gift and trust from God. It is not mine to dispose of at my own behest. Rather, I am to use it faithfully, subject to God's authority; and I am answerable to God beyond this life for the way that I do use it. Moreover, God promises to uphold me in his care through whatever I have to endure in this life, and there may be redemptive possibilities hidden in the darkest episodes I have yet to face." Anyone can see that these different commitments could very naturally lead to very different positions concerning the permissibility of voluntary euthanasia. Indeed, one of the reasons why the question of euthanasia can appear to be so intractable when it is debated in the public arena is, I think, that the various positions in the debate may spring from very different fundamental convictions of those kinds – convictions which are hardly likely to be overturned or even modified during a public discussion of a medical ethical question.

An adequately deep and properly comprehensive treatment of the question of euthanasia would explore that whole terrain of issues. But I am going to try to keep the huge world-view issues to the side, at least for the time being. I am going to persist in my attempt to concentrate on common moral ground, and to see whether it can provide an adequate basis for some resolution of the problem of euthanasia. I will suggest a line of thought which proceeds in a fairly simple way from the kinds of attitudes and principles to which members of the caring professions have already committed themselves, including the four-principles framework. Let us see whether this line of thought helps us to attain some genuine ethical clarity on the question.

If we are working with our ordinary and uncontroversial principles of medical ethics, we can state the case *for* voluntary active euthanasia by means of a straightforward appeal to both beneficence and autonomy. The argument from beneficence would stress that, when a person is suffering terribly, and his suffering will end only, sooner or later, in death, the *good* that we owe him is release from that suffering. It may be the case that we can diminish his suffering through palliation; but this will still involve prolonged suffering, albeit at a lower level. The good that we owe him is the *minimisation* of his suffering, and this requires the swiftest, surest release. Hence euthanasia. The argument from autonomy would stress that this release is precisely what the patient *wants*: he has expressly requested it. If we are to give due regard to what he wishes, if we really *respect* him as a *person*, then we will be governed by what he wants. It is his life, and his death, not ours. The right to decide what happens to him is *his* right. Hence euthanasia.

The weight of the case for voluntary active euthanasia, then, is the accumulated weight of those two arguments. If one seeks to rebut those arguments by appeal to the principle of non-maleficence, by saying that to kill the patient would be to breach this principle because it would entail doing terrible *harm* to the patient, then the proponent of euthanasia can respond that this is a mistake. For, he can say, the harm that matters is the patient's suffering. And because all that is now left for the patient is a period of suffering, our duty is to release him from that harm. Killing, in this situation, does not cause harm: it minimises harm. So it would be no breach of our duty of non-maleficence.

We also often hear, as part of the case for euthanasia, an appeal to the *dignity* of the patient, and the notion of dignity here can be linked either to beneficence, or to autonomy, or to both. The connection with beneficence is made when we claim that a person who is suffering the ravages of a terminal illness is a person whose dignity is thereby undermined – so that a restoration of dignity would require a release from that degradation and suffering. The connection with autonomy is made when we claim that we are not treating a person with dignity, we are not fully respecting him as a person, when we override his own wishes. For either or both of these reasons, then, it is claimed that voluntary active euthanasia provides *death with dignity*.

I do not think that we can take a serious part in this discussion unless we feel the very great weight behind those arguments. Experienced healthcare professionals do not require any fertility of imagination to depict for themselves a patient racked by what can be the appalling pain and frightful degradation of terminal illness. Anyone who can stand by the bedside of such a patient and *not* wish for his swift release from that condition is a person devoid of human compassion.

But does this mean that the arguments for voluntary active euthanasia carry the day?

To try to answer the question of whether those arguments are successful, I want to take a small step to the side, and consider for a little while a slightly different, but importantly related, kind of situation. I propose that we perform a short case study. I have taken the case from *Modern Medicine of South Africa*, where it was used as part of a questionnaire surveying South African doctors' attitudes on issues concerning the end of life. Since June 1992, when it appeared in the magazine, I have used the case in my courses for medical students and in discussions with various colleagues in the healthcare professions. It is as follows:

> A 36-year-old man with AIDS has a history of several painful opportunistic infections that were resolved with great difficulty. Upon being discharged from the hospital following an episode of influenza, the patient asks for a prescription for an analgesic narcotic, a syringe, and information as to what dosages would result in death. He has put his affairs in order and executed all legal documents. It is understood, though not spoken, that the patient intends suicide.

It is important to note that this case was first published before anti-retroviral medications opened up the possibility of good long-term management of HIV patients. It will be helpful for the purposes of our discussion if we think of the case as it was in those days (and would still be in the many parts of the world in which anti-retroviral medication is unavailable) – that is, as a case of terminal illness.

What is at issue in this case is, of course, physician-assisted suicide. I find that the very general response to this case, both among students and among practising professionals, is that it would be wrong for the doctor to give this man what he is asking for. This is a response I share. Yet precisely parallel arguments to those we heard in support of voluntary active euthanasia – the arguments from beneficence and autonomy – can be mounted in support of physician-assisted suicide in this case. It can be claimed that this man is facing a terrible future of decline caused by his terminal illness – a future of great suffering, perhaps magnified by loneliness and desolation. The *good* we owe him is release from this future. It can also be claimed that this release is quite clearly what he *wants*, and that we ought to be governed by what he wants. How, then, can we feel that we ought not to assist his suicide? In the face of those clear and forceful arguments to the contrary, where does our very general response come from?

Let us look a little more closely at those arguments for assisting the man to kill himself, and let us start with the argument from autonomy. Do we feel that it applies as well to suicide in general? Do we feel that we ought to assist anyone who wants to commit suicide? Certainly not. We commonly take for granted not only that we are entitled to withhold our assistance, but also that we may actively intervene to *prevent* suicide. Popular culture – represented by books, films, and so on – demonstrates this assumption frequently: it often portrays as *heroic* the person who is prepared to intervene to prevent an attempted suicide.

And if we are entitled to prevent suicide, then we are even more clearly entitled *not to assist* it. So the argument from autonomy would be giving us the wrong moral answer in the case of suicide in general. (In some jurisdictions, suicide is not *illegal*, but that certainly does not entail that we have a *moral* duty to *assist* it.)

Now if we were pressed to justify this common assumption concerning suicide, we might go on to point out that the suicidal desire can be reversed. Most persons who attempt suicide but are saved do not go on to commit suicide later: they apparently do not persist in their wish to die. And this surely supports our assumption that we are entitled to intervene.

However, someone might appeal to that very fact *in support* of the argument from autonomy. For – they might say – if the wish to die is reversible, then it is not the person's *true* wish; it must rather be a mere cry for help, or the symptom of some temporary emotional or mental disturbance. And so it will not, in such a case, be the person's *genuinely autonomous* wish: it will not be the true wish of a person fully in possession of himself. But then it is unsurprising that we are entitled to intervene to prevent his suicide, for we are thereby stopping him from doing what he does not truly, genuinely wish to do. In intervening, we are acting *consistently* with what his genuinely autonomous wish would be. In other words, we are in fact governed by the autonomy principle. But then, *by the same principle*, if a person really *does*, genuinely autonomously, wish to die, then we are required to assist him to do so.

But I reject that line of reasoning. There are no doubt many cases of attempted suicide in which the wish to die is not fully genuine. But there are no doubt also many cases in which the wish to die *is* quite genuine and serious, *and* in which it can be reversed. How can it be reversed? Many attempted suicides lose their wish to die in response to the care shown towards them by others. It is not that their wish would not have persisted had their situation remained as it was. It is that the new factor in their lives, the care shown by others, actually alters their assessment of their own worth. For the attempted suicide's self-assessment is typically that his life – he himself – has no worth, or potential worth. Hence his despair, his sense of desolation. But the care he then receives – care offered by others who *recognise his value as a person* – demonstrates that his life *is* worthwhile, and that it *was* at least potentially worthwhile. Indeed, his desperate, suicidal wish might have been due, at least in some part, to a lack of provision of that life-enriching care by those in some way or another related to him. And this surely indicates our highest moral duty to the attempted suicide. Our responsibility is to offer the care that will demonstrate that his life, he himself, is worthwhile. And where we can do this, we do not fulfil our duty towards him, but rather fail in that duty when we accede to his wish to die.

Grant Gillett helpfully reviews various motivations which may drive a person towards suicide, and argues that each such kind of case presents to the rest of us a challenge which "is captured by the question 'How did we fail you?'"[8] How are we to show to this person the care that will reverse the suicidal desire?

So much for suicide in general. But the AIDS patient in our case study is not just any person harbouring a suicidal wish: he is terminally ill. What difference does this make to our duty towards him? It is arguable that it makes little or no difference. For we can readily imagine – and I think it is this that largely gives rise to our intuitive response to the case – that this young man is suffering a sense of hopelessness and desolation, a sense of worthlessness, which is very like that suffered by attempted suicides in general. He may well feel that he is now staring into the abyss of the disintegration of his life, of his very self. The prospect of unrelieved and progressive suffering may be accompanied by a terrible sense of personal isolation. The stigma attached to AIDS, his possible rejection by those close to him, a possible sense of shame or guilt concerning his disease – all these can produce an acute form of that sense of desolation or worthlessness which is typical of suicides in general. And *we* need not merely *enquire* how we can provide the kind of care that will reverse his suicidal wish: we already *know* that there is much that we can do. We can promise him a commitment of medical care which will effectively manage the symptoms of his progressive illness. We can come alongside him with a commitment of real personal support – the kind of support which allows him to air his feelings of despair, and which provides the very thing that dispels them. Once again, this is surely where our real moral duty to him lies.

Now we have arrived at this conclusion by pursuing a line of thought which began with our considering the argument from autonomy – the argument that we should assist him to commit suicide because this is what he expressly requests. And our conclusion provides us with an answer to that argument. The argument appeals to what the patient *wants*. But as we analyse that want, and what gives rise to it, we see that its very existence indicates a failure of, or at least the need for, *care* on our part. So our acceding to what he wants would be inconsistent with our duty of care towards him. Our duty, rather, is to provide the very care that will dispel the want.

However, there was also the argument from beneficence – the argument that we ought to assist his suicide because it would be for his good to be released from his future of suffering.

But our answer to the argument from autonomy also provides us with an answer to this argument from beneficence. For what we have seen entails that the greatest good that we can provide for him is the life-enriching care to which we have been referring – the care that will show him that his life, that he himself, has worth and value, even through the process of his dying. Far from serving his good, then, we would be helping to extinguish what is of real value if we were to assist him to hasten his death by his own hand.

Now, how does that case study help us to respond to those arguments for voluntary active euthanasia which we heard earlier? The connection is this, and it is crucial: the testimony of those who care well for dying patients indicates that a desire for euthanasia is – typically, and very importantly – similar to the kind of suicidal desire that we have been considering. For terminal illness can produce a sense of desolation and worthlessness very similar to that suffered by suicidal persons. In terminal illness, many of the props which ordinarily support our sense of the worthwhileness of life fall away. Again, Gillett helpfully diagnoses the kind of state of mind which can arise in a patient facing death, "the great unknown":

> At the moment of death a person quits all that is familiar… What is clear is that there is a final break with the relationships and everyday familiar things which fill the hours and days of human life. In the face of this unknown, many people need support and reassurance that they are not being abandoned. The feeling of being discarded or passed over as no longer of any worth is, it seems, one of the worst aspects of dying for many patients.[9]

And where this state of mind arises, it is surely the duty of the rest of us to provide that support and reassurance to which Gillett refers – the personal support and care which affirm the worth of the patient and his life, even through the process of his dying, and which are, in this respect, just like the support and care we owe to the suicidal person.

But as I say, the evidence of those with relevant experience is that a request for euthanasia typically occurs when that kind of committed personal care is absent, and very often falls away when the care is present. Members of the hospice movement and others who practise expert palliative medicine report that very few, if any, patients have untreatable pain. The pain and other distressing symptoms of terminal illness, they tell us, can almost always be managed at a tolerable level by good palliative medicine. And interestingly enough, it is not those patients with the least manageable symptoms who issue a request for euthanasia. Rather, the request seems typically to arise from that sense of despair and worthlessness we have noted – a sense which can be dispelled by real personal support and care.[10]

This is tremendously interesting testimony from the experts in palliative care, for it strongly suggests that the desire for euthanasia should be presumed to belong in the same category as the desire for suicide, in the respects that we considered earlier. And if this is the case, then our moral response to a request for euthanasia ought to be parallel to our moral response to a request for assistance in suicide. In particular, our answers to the arguments for assistance in suicide ought to provide parallel answers to the arguments for voluntary active euthanasia.

Thus, the argument from autonomy would be answered in the following way. We ought not to be governed by the *request* for euthanasia. For the want embodied in this request is a want which is itself due to our failure of care, or which at least indicates the need for our care – care which, when provided, can be expected to dispel the want. By contrast, if we were to accede to the request for euthanasia, we would in effect be endorsing the underlying sense of worthlessness, the underlying self-rejection, from which it springs. And what a tragic irony this would involve if the sense of despair were due to our failure of care in the first place! What is at stake here is the contest between what are *in effect* two utterly different attitudes towards the patient. On the one hand: "You regard yourself as no longer of any worth. We agree. Here, be our guest. End it all." On the other hand: "You may *feel* yourself to be worthless, but we attach great value to you. And we want to demonstrate your value by our care for you."

Similarly, the argument from beneficence would also be answered by what we have said in response to the argument from autonomy. We do not act for the patient's good in killing him; instead, we extinguish a life, a person, who is still of value. The care that we owe him is genuinely *life-enriching*; and it is the felt enrichment provided by that care which serves to overturn the patient's desire for a premature, unnatural death. Those committed to caring well for the terminally ill testify to the many ways in which patients supported by that personal care can find the last stages of their life intensely valuable and significant.

It was presumably for these reasons that Dame Cicely Saunders, pioneer of the hospice movement, said that euthanasia "should be unnecessary and is an admission of defeat".[11] It should be unnecessary because good palliative medicine can provide the relief which the patient needs. It is an admission of defeat because it would occur at the patient's request only when he has not received the care and support which we ought to provide for him – the care and support that would displace his request for euthanasia.

Our responses to the arguments from autonomy and beneficence also provide us with an answer to the appeal to the dignity of the patient. We can now claim that it is not euthanasia which provides death with dignity. The dying patient is accorded his true dignity not when his death is hastened by a false sense of his worthlessness, but when his genuine value as a person is honoured through the real care and support provided to him.

So our answers to those arguments suggest a general moral conclusion concerning voluntary active euthanasia. Euthanasia is not where the healthcare professional's duty lies. It would seem, indeed, to be *contrary* to our duty to the terminally ill: our duty is to provide these patients with good palliative medicine and genuine personal support. Thus we arrive at a conclusion which sits quite comfortably within the traditional medical ethos. This is not merely because medical ethics has traditionally viewed euthanasia with disapproval; it is because at the heart of the medical ethos lies a commitment of *care* for the patient – of care which is offered without regard to the relative value of the patient's life; of care *especially* for sub-optimal life, for life which is tenuous, for life which is passing away. And our duty of care is exactly that: a duty to *care*, not a duty to despatch.

This duty of care will, of course, be distributed across the healthcare *team* (including social workers and others), for not every member of the team will have the time or possess the particular clinical medical expertise or the special personal skills and sensitivities required to provide the expert palliative care and support needed by the terminally ill. What is obviously required is an exercise of interdisciplinary teamwork.

This suggested conclusion concerning voluntary active euthanasia gives us consequent conclusions concerning the other species of euthanasia. If voluntary active euthanasia is impermissible, then involuntary and non-voluntary active euthanasia are even more clearly impermissible. The same can be said for passive euthanasia, where this would involve withholding some treatment which would support life and which would be owed as part of the normal duty of care – except for the following qualification. The extent to which we can *impose* treatment, even life-sustaining treatment, upon the patient is severely constrained by what the patient wants. As we noted in Chapter Five, in a case where a patient adamantly and consistently refuses treatment, the healthcare professionals *may*, in the end, sadly have to accept his refusal. And this means that, in principle, we may have to acquiesce in what is effectively the patient's suicide. We could call this a case of voluntary passive euthanasia but for the fact that we would not be *seeking* the patient's death; hence it is better not to call it euthanasia at all.

In this way, it seems to me, we reach a proper general conclusion about euthanasia for healthcare ethics. Euthanasia ought not to be accepted as a legitimate option within medical practice.

This case against euthanasia has been centred upon our duty of care to the patient, understood by reference to the four principles. But it can be reinforced by various further arguments. Many of those who are opposed to euthanasia draw our attention to what they say would be the *bad consequences* of accepting it as a legitimate medical option. As we noted in Chapter Four, it is not only the consequentialist who is interested in consequences; the non-consequentialist can also insist that we take into account the consequences of an action or policy. And many commentators believe that euthanasia is a case in which the consequences can in fact decide the ethical issue. They argue that even if it were true that certain particular *acts* of euthanasia would be morally permissible, it is also true that a *policy* of allowing euthanasia would carry the risk of various bad consequences, and that these risks are serious enough to render such a policy irresponsible, even if the policy provided permission for only voluntary euthanasia under stringent conditions. The concerns of these commentators are widely discussed, and I shall not take the space to review them in detail here. But I believe that they deserve to be mentioned briefly.

Some commentators seek to raise the spectre of Hitler and the Holocaust, pointing to the horrors of the Nazi "euthanasia" programme, and claiming that we would be in danger of going in the same direction if we permitted euthanasia as a medical practice. Now it is easy to regard such a claim as badly unjustified – perhaps even hysterical. For the kind of euthanasia called for by its contemporary advocates in the Western world is voluntary euthanasia, the practice of which would be subject to strict conditions, and this is hardly on a par with what was done under the Nazi programme. All the same, the thoughtful commentators who believe that we ought to take careful note of what happened under the Nazis are concerned about the kind of slippery slope which can open out when the *attitudes* of healthcare professionals shift in such a way as to embrace the possibility of euthanasia. When the caring professions accept that there is such a thing as a life not worth living, what kinds of patients, what kinds of persons, might eventually be included within that category? And when the normal social and psychological barrier against killing is removed through a "medicalization of killing", where might the killing policy eventually lead? These were the beginnings of the German medical profession's collaboration in mass murder.[12] Can we confidently calculate that, despite the same shift in basic attitudes, other doctors and carers would not slide into some relevantly similar kind of abyss?

There are very real concerns about the possibilities of *abuse* of a policy permitting euthanasia. For instance, might patients be killed, or allowed to die, when it is not (as the policy would require it to be) for *their good*? As Philippa Foot remarks:

> Many people want, and want very badly, to be rid of their elderly relatives and even of their ailing husbands or wives. Would any safeguards ever be able to stop them describing as euthanasia what was really for their own benefit?[13]

Or might patients be killed, or allowed to die, when it is not (as the policy would require it to be) what *they want?* Might non-voluntary (and perhaps even involuntary) euthanasia be tolerated and practised?

I have referred to these as concerns about the *possibility* of abuse of a policy permissive of voluntary euthanasia. But in fact, a number of studies of actual practice within jurisdictions in which voluntary euthanasia is permitted (e.g. the Netherlands) at least appear to indicate that these various kinds of abuse *have* occurred.[14]

There is also the concern that, under a policy permitting euthanasia, some patients may issue a request for euthanasia not because this is what they really want, but because they feel some, supposed or real, pressure from elsewhere – for instance, pressure from their family or others shouldering the burden of care or paying the medical bills; pressure from their medical aid scheme; pressure from the hospital providing their care; and so on. Pressure can, of course, be subtle yet effective. In other words, what would *look* like voluntary euthanasia would not be truly voluntary.

Furthermore, we might be concerned that a policy permitting euthanasia would diminish patients' trust in their doctors and hospitals – the trust on which good healthcare so critically relies. Many members of the public, particularly in developing countries, operate with a relatively unsophisticated understanding of healthcare policy. For these laypersons, the fact that doctors are known to be killers as well as sustainers of life might well cause a real loss of trust, which would, in turn, undermine the effectiveness of the provisions for healthcare.

And finally, such a policy could alter, very much for the worse, our general attitudes towards the elderly and towards the chronically ill or disabled; and it could similarly alter those persons' attitudes towards themselves. Again, Philippa Foot:

> … the possibility of active voluntary euthanasia might change the social scene in ways that would be very bad. As things are, people do, by and large, expect to be looked after if they are old or ill. This is one of the good things that we have, but we might lose it, and be much worse off without it. It might come to be expected that someone likely to need a lot of looking after should call for the doctor and demand his own death. Something comparable could be good in an extremely poverty-stricken community where the children genuinely suffered from lack of food; but in rich societies such as ours it would surely be a spiritual disaster. Such possibilities should make us very wary of supporting large measures of euthanasia, even where moral principle applied to the individual act does not rule it out.[15]

It seems to me that these various considerations converge towards the conclusion that the healthcare professions are wise to maintain their traditional prohibition of euthanasia. There is considerable debate about the likelihood of those bad consequences we have just reviewed. But it is plausible to hold that each is accompanied by some substantial likelihood; and each consequence, if it occurred, would be seriously bad. It would seem to follow, then, that we ought not to risk those consequences. Now, of course, there are many situations where we are entitled to risk some bad consequence because this cannot be avoided while we are pursuing some important good. (The ambulance drives at high speed, thereby risking an accident on the road, because of the urgent need to get the patient to the emergency department.) But our earlier case against euthanasia showed that the duty of care towards the patient is properly discharged without the option of euthanasia. So we do not *need* to risk these bad consequences in order to provide the best care for our patients: these risks are not the unfortunate but inevitable risks attached to the pursuit of an important good. And if they are risks that we *need not* bring about, then they are risks that we *ought not* to bring about.

Thus, our earlier conclusion that euthanasia is impermissible is reinforced by these concerns about the bad consequences of a policy permitting euthanasia.

As I pointed out, this conclusion fits comfortably within traditional medical ethics. Over some decades, I have been discussing this issue with professional groups, and I have found that the line of thought which leads to this conclusion – the line of thought which stresses our duty of committed care – has been very generally endorsed by the members of those groups, whatever their own personal world-view commitments. Nevertheless, it is a conclusion, and line of thought, which is increasingly challenged by campaigns for the legalisation of euthanasia, which in some jurisdictions have recently been successful. If the line of thought pursued in this chapter is sound, then our duty of care does not require the option of euthanasia. What *is* needed is adequate provision for proper palliative care, but not euthanasia. But this does not satisfy some of the campaigners. They would insist that, despite my claim to pay due heed to the principle of autonomy, the line of thought I have advocated does not take sufficiently seriously their demand to be allowed to determine for themselves the conditions under which they shall continue to live and the conditions under which they can choose to die.

Many of those campaigners claim that traditional medical ethics is blocking their way because it stands in thrall to old religious prejudices. They feel that the traditional medical ethos has been unduly influenced by a theistic world-view, which has imported into medicine a cluster of distortions – a mystical reverence for mere human life, however lacking in quality this life might be; an unreasonable prohibition of killing; and an infantile attitude to individual human autonomy. "It is *my* life that we are talking about, and it is *my* right to choose the conditions under which my life is to continue," the campaigners would insist. "Medical ethics needs to be liberated from old superstitions. It needs to be reformed."

In pursuing the line of thought I have advocated, I tried to put the contest between world-views to the side, and to see what progress we could make on the basis of common ground. But the campaigners whose protest we have just heard will feel that, in failing to provide space for their much more radical demand for autonomy, I have failed to find adequate common ground. I am, they would say, excluding concerns which are central to their naturalistic picture of the world.

We have here a reminder that we would be foolish to ignore the fact that in discussing these issues, we may find ourselves caught up into the clash between very different world-views.

And in the next chapter, we will see that clash brought into considerably sharper relief.

Notes

1 Earlier versions of the substance of much of this chapter were presented in my articles "On Euthanasia", in M.D. Smith, D. Pantanowitz and G. J. Oettle, Eds., *Surgical Oncology: Proceedings of the 18th Biennial Congress of the Department of Surgery, University of the Witwatersrand*, June 2001, pp. 145–54; and "Euthanasia: A Problem for Psychiatrists", in *South African Psychiatry Review*, Vol. 7, No. 1, February 2004, pp. 10–18.

2 Philippa Foot, "Euthanasia", in her *Virtues and Vices* (Blackwell, Oxford, 1978), pp. 33–61.

3 I have discussed these limits in my "Thinking about the Living Will", *South African Medical Journal*, Vol. 85, No. 11, November 1995, pp. 1146–7.

4 Grant Gillett, *Reasonable Care* (Bristol Press, Bristol, 1989), Chapter 4. As will be seen below, I have found this chapter and Chapter 6 of Gillett's book to be particularly helpful in this general discussion. I commend those chapters to the reader.

5 The origin of this "15th Century folk-saying" is apparently unknown. (Quentin Shaw, "On Aphorisms", *British Journal of General Practice*, 2009 Dec. 1; 59 (569): pp. 954–5.) Nevertheless, it is variously attributed to Ambroise Paré, Edward Livingston Trudeau, and Hippocrates.

6 Some philosophically trained readers will wonder whether I ought to have put an "only if" in this statement of the criterion, and in the previously stated proportionality criterion. But they will quickly recognise the complicated reasons why I prefer to leave the criteria roughly stated. I am not attempting to provide a set of individually necessary and jointly sufficient conditions of the moral permissibility of, respectively, ceasing to pursue the good and pursuing the good.

7 David Atkinson, *Pastoral Ethics in Practice*, (Monarch, Eastbourne, 1989), p. 228.

8 Gillett, *op.cit.*, p. 98.

9 *Ibid.*, p. 95.

10 Cf., e.g., Gillett, *ibid.* p. 99; Elizabeth J. Latimer, "Euthanasia: A Physician's Reflections", *Journal of Pain and Symptom Management*, Vol. 6, No. 8, November 1991, pp. 487–91, at p. 488; Elizabeth J. Latimer and James McGregor, "Euthanasia, physician-assisted suicide and the ethical care of dying patients", *Canadian Medical Association Journal*, 1994; 151 (8), pp. 1133–36, at p. 1134; Roger Woodruff, "Euthanasia and Physician-Assisted Suicide – Are They Clinically Necessary?", *International Association for Hospice and Palliative Care*, 1999, at http://hospicecare.com/resources/ethical-issues/essays-and-articles-on-ethics-in-palliative-care/euthanasia-and-physician-assisted-suicide-are-they-clinically-necessary/; Lukas Radbruch *et al*, "Euthanasia and physician-assisted suicide: A white paper from the European Association for Palliative Care", *Palliative Medicine*, 2015, at http://journals.sagepub.com/doi/abs/10.1177/0269216315616524?legid=sppmj%3B0269216315616524v1&patientinform-links=yes

11 Quoted in Jonathan Glover, *Causing Death and Saving Lives*, (Penguin, Harmondsworth, 1977), p. 190.

12 Beauchamp and Childress, *op. cit.*, 4th edition, (1994), pp. 231–2.

13 *Op.cit.*, p. 58.

14 These studies are reviewed by Woodruff, *op. cit.*, and Radbruch *et al*, *op. cit.* The studies are discussed by Charles Camosy: "Right to Die, or Duty to Die? The Slippery-Slope Argument Against Euthanasia Revisited", at www.abc.net.au/religion/articles/2014/09/01/4078456.htm

15 *Op. cit.*, p. 59.

7
Disability, screening, and the value of human life

In this final chapter, I want to discuss an issue which arises in every caring profession: what is our duty of care towards people with disability? There are two reasons why I select this as our final topic. First, in considering this issue, we shall have a good deal of room to continue to practise the application of the material we gathered in the first part of the book. However, it will be important for us to recognise that on this issue, we can receive only *limited* help from some of that material, for we have now arrived in deeply contested territory. I will persist in my appeal to our common moral sense. But we shall hear our common-sense views being attacked head-on, particularly from one kind of philosophical theory. We shall see that the four principles are insufficient to guide our way out of this clash. And we shall be unable to dodge the conflict between different world-views. We shall find, though, that we have plenty of scope to apply our tools of critical reasoning. The second reason for selecting this issue is that, while wrestling our way through this disputed territory, we shall be asking what are perhaps the most *basic* ethical questions about the nature of our duty of care. Is it a duty that we owe to all persons equally, or are some human lives more valuable than others? For we shall find that there is a vital connection between the question of our duty of care for the disabled and those fundamental questions concerning the value of human life.

Attitudes to disability

When we turn to consider our treatment of the disabled, it is quickly obvious that two very noticeable developments have taken place over the last few decades.

The first of these developments has occurred in our change of attitude towards disabled people. Very considerable efforts have been made, at least in Western countries, to bring into the mainstream of society those whose lives would, a

DOI: 10.4324/9781003176541-9

few decades ago, have been largely confined to institutions. We are learning to listen to the disabled, to recognise the value of their lives, and to understand their needs. In particular, we are learning how to remove the barriers which stand in the way of their full participation in society. Workplaces are now designed to accommodate disabled staff and customers. Laws have been introduced to ensure that employment and insurance arrangements do not discriminate against the disabled. Disabled people are honoured within our cultural activities. Some appear as presenters on our television screens. We celebrate their achievements on the sporting field, in the Paralympics and similar events. In these and other ways, the social stigma attached to disability is being removed, and the lives of the disabled are being respected and appreciated. Advocates for the disabled point out that much more can yet be done, but real strides have already been taken.

But over the same period, another very marked trend has been occurring within the healthcare professions. Various pre-natal tests have been developed which can detect some problems before or during pregnancy. Some of these tests can be of great help in ensuring that the health of the mother or of the developing baby is protected. But much testing is done in order to detect abnormality in the embryo or foetus – abnormality which would result in disability of some kind. This testing is becoming more and more widespread. In many places, it is now routine. And when an abnormality is detected, the standard practice is to abort the pregnancy.

Anyone can see the tension – indeed, the apparent contradiction – between these two developments. On the one hand, we have been taking some pains to respect the disabled, to value their lives, and to welcome them into the mainstream of society. On the other hand, we are busily eliminating them in the earliest stages of their development.

Members of the caring professions are deeply involved on both sides of this tension. They lead the way in the care and promotion of disabled people within society. They also lead the way in the elimination of the lives of disabled people before birth. Is this moral schizophrenia? Are these the Jekyll and Hyde faces of the caring professions? How should we be thinking about this?

Screening

The various procedures used in pre-natal testing are commonly referred to together under the general term "screening", and give rise to what is in fact a complex mix of ethical questions. The main question concerns *the point* of screening. I have mentioned that some tests have an important therapeutic purpose: they provide vital information that assists the medical team to protect the health and safety of mother and developing child. But many of the disorders which screening seeks to detect are conditions for which there is no cure or therapy. In some cases, the information that the foetus carries this condition may provide knowledge which assists the medical team to manage the pregnancy more carefully; and it may assist the parents to prepare for the care, or the adoption, of their disabled child. But in most of these cases, the information is sought in order to decide whether to terminate the pregnancy. My medical colleagues tell me that in the vast majority of the cases in which some disorder is detected, abortion is indeed chosen. This is called selective abortion because its purpose is to prevent the birth of a baby with the detected disorder. The main point of screening is a decision concerning selective abortion (or the discarding of the embryo, in those cases in which it is fertilised and tested *in vitro*). Is this morally justified?

More specifically, if our purpose is a decision concerning selective abortion, are we justified in screening for the *particular* conditions for which screening is, or can be, performed? Screening can detect conditions which result in extreme disability, or great suffering for the disabled child, and which can impose an enormous burden of care upon the parents of the disabled offspring and create huge consequences for their families. Other detectable disorders (e.g., Down's syndrome, or some instances of spina bifida) are much less severe; though it must be noted that the same condition may be regarded as severe by some people, but as not severe by others. Some of the detectable disorders can be surgically repaired or treated after birth. And some of these disorders cause very minor disabilities, such as cleft lip or club foot. Screening can detect some conditions which will cause illness or disability or death only once the offspring has advanced well into adult life. It can detect the sex of the foetus (thus providing information desired by those parents who wish only for a girl, or only for a boy, and which is particularly desired in those countries in which male children are strongly preferred). And so on. Are medical professionals morally justified in offering screening for *all* these conditions, and should parents be entitled to use screening in order to be able to choose abortion in all these cases?

I have been talking as if screening straightforwardly detects the conditions it is looking for; but in fact, matters are not so simple, and the complexities here raise further ethical problems. Many of the screening tests indicate only a risk, a *probability*, that the foetus carries the condition in question; and it can be very difficult to interpret the significance of such a probability, if indeed we properly understand in the first place that it is a mere probability. Many tests have significant false positive or false negative rates. That is to say, in a significant number of cases they indicate that the disorder being tested for is present even though it is not in fact present, or that it is absent in cases where it is in fact present. And some of the most reliable, directly diagnostic tests are invasive, and in a significant number of cases they cause complications, including miscarriage. (So, for instance, a pregnant mother may be offered a test for foetal abnormality in a case where the probability of an abnormality is comparable to the probability of miscarriage due to the test, and thus where the chance that an abnormality will be discovered by the test is roughly the same as the chance that the test will itself cause the abortion of a normal pregnancy.) The upshot of all this is that normal pregnancies can be aborted even after testing for abnormality and even when the parents would have preferred to have the baby if they had known that it was normal. Medical colleagues report that many of these cases do in fact occur. (It is easy to see how this could happen. Suppose that we terminate each pregnancy in which the chance of some abnormality is, say, one in two. Then roughly half of all the foetuses we abort will be normal. If our test for this abnormality has a significant false positivity rate, then that will tend to raise further the number of normal foetuses we abort. If the test has a significant miscarriage rate, then a number of abortions of normal foetuses will be caused by the test itself…) And no doubt some abnormal pregnancies proceed to term even after testing and even when the parents would have wanted to choose abortion if they had known of the abnormality. (Perhaps the parents bet against an outcome that carries a low probability. Perhaps the test returns a false negative result…) These facts serve to reinforce our concerns as to whether the screening process is justified. Furthermore, they underline for us how important it is that prospective parents *understand* the unreliabilities and uncertainties attached to screening, so that they are in a position to give truly *informed consent* to the various steps in the process. Many genetic counsellors take pains to ensure that parents are properly informed, but they voice their worries as to whether they manage to succeed. And of course, it needs to be understood that screening can offer no guarantee that the baby will be normal and healthy; for, quite apart from the uncertainties within the testing process, there are many disorders for which there is no pre-natal test.

But at the heart of this cluster of issues is the question I raised at the outset: should we be choosing between lives in this kind of way? Ought we to regard a life of disability as a life we can dispense with; as a life not requiring the kind of care and support that we provide to normal lives?

Our current practices take for granted that we are entitled to use screening for this purpose. Some people, in fact, argue that parents *should* use screening and selective abortion in order to do their best to have normal children rather than disabled children.[1]

But it is hardly surprising that many disabled people themselves find this offensive. They feel that it represents a wrong kind of discrimination against the disabled – the very discrimination which contemporary societies have been trying to undo, in the workplace, in cultural life, and so on. Advocates for the disabled stress how valuable the lives of the disabled can be; and they argue that we are therefore wrong in eliminating these lives in favour of normal lives.

Now it seems to me that advocates for the disabled sometimes over-state their case. In their effort to stress the value of the lives of the disabled, they sometimes insist that there is nothing wrong with, or bad about, disability; it is just different. The problems faced by disabled people, they say, are not problems concerning the condition of their bodies. They are social problems. The real problem is to remove the barriers which society has placed in the way of their full participation in society. They do not need their bodies to be "fixed"; they need the social barriers to be removed. Disability ought to be regarded simply as part of the diversity to be welcomed in society.

And such advocates would object to my description of the conditions which can cause disability (the conditions which screening seeks to detect). It is not right to describe these conditions as "abnormal", they say. This kind of description simply reinforces the social stigma attached to disability, which obstructs the proper inclusion of disabled people within mainstream society. It represents a wrongly discriminatory attitude towards the disabled – an attitude which deserves to be called "able-ism" (on a parallel with racism or sexism). Once again, there is nothing abnormal about disability; it is just different.

But this, as I say, seems to me to over-state the case. If it were true that there is nothing bad or wrong or undesirable about disability – nothing that we ought to regard as regrettable, or unfortunate – then all the medical textbooks would need to be rewritten. For the terms they use to describe the conditions which cause disability have an essentially *evaluative* element. The textbooks talk not only of *abnormalities*, but also of genetic *diseases* and *disorders*; of genetic or congenital *errors*; of developmental *defects*; of *dysfunction*; of *handicaps*, and so on. All these terms imply that something is not as it ought to be; and if this implication is incorrect, then the terms must be replaced with different terms that carry no such implication. But the view that there is nothing bad about disability has an even more untenable consequence. If this view were true, then a parent who *causes* disability in an ordinary (normal) child would be doing no harm. If a parent (or anyone else, for that matter) blinded a sighted child, or deafened a hearing child, or caused in a normal child spina bifida, or Down's syndrome, then he or she would not be harming the child or doing anything bad to it. The parent would simply be making the child different, but not in such a way that makes the child worse off. And this is surely an utterly unacceptable consequence of the view. Any parent who did such a thing would be doing grievous harm to the child, and acting very wrongly indeed.

The word "disability" itself has an evaluative implication. It suggests to us that the person who is disabled has been *deprived* of an ability that we would typically expect. And thus it suggests to us what is bad about the relevant underlying condition (the kind of condition that screening seeks to detect). The condition deprives the person of an ability by impeding the proper *function* of some part of the human body. And a loss of bodily function, and consequent loss of ability, typically makes that human worse off. However, we do not need to deny this fact about disability in order to affirm the value of the lives of people who live with a disability. They themselves stress how rich their lives can be, and how much they can enjoy and offer – particularly if we do not exclude them from the range of interactions and activities available in mainstream society.

And while accepting that disability does typically make the disabled person worse off, we can also recognise how our practices of screening and selective abortion are felt as reinforcing the discrimination against disabled people. How can we be selectively destroying the disabled in the earliest stages of their development unless we regard their lives as less valuable than those of normal people? If we thought that disability made life so bad that it would be better for the disabled person to have no life at all, then we might claim that in aborting the disabled, we are acting in *their* best interests. But – with the exception of a few extreme conditions – we do not believe that disability makes life as bad as that. So doesn't our practice of selective abortion in fact show that we believe that the disabled are not owed the same care as normal people?

Disabled people often testify that the very discussion of screening can make them feel that their lives are indeed being devalued in this way. And they report that they are exposed to offensive remarks to this effect. Here is one example, reported by the late Stella Young, an Australian writer, comedian, and disability activist:

> A few years ago I was approached by a nervous looking woman on a tram on my way home from work. "Excuse me," she said. "Do you have Osteogenesis Imperfecta?" With a friendly tone, I confirmed that I do. Most of the time when people are specific with the name of a relatively rare condition like mine, it's because they know someone else with it. So I was surprised by her next line. "I was pregnant with a baby with OI and I had a termination." I nodded, but let that sentence hang in the air between us for a moment. My throat had tightened and I didn't quite trust myself to speak. It was she who broke the silence for us both. Looking me directly in the eye, she took a deep breath and said, "I made the right decision." Then she got off the tram.[2]

Those of us who do not live with disability can only imagine how hurtful – and indeed threatening – such remarks and attitudes must be.[3]

Advocates for the disabled point out that such attitudes arise when we see only *the condition* that causes the disability, and not *the person* who happens to carry that condition. If we were to see the person, we would recognise that he or she is indeed a person just like the rest of us – at least in those respects which touch upon our value as persons. Consequently, disability advocates urge us to think and talk of *people with a disability*, not of *the disabled*, or even of *disabled people*.

But interestingly enough, that very same distinction – between person and condition – is appealed to by those who defend screening against the charge that it reinforces discrimination against the disabled. They claim that screening seeks to prevent *the condition*; it does *not* devalue *the person*. Here is how the American medical ethicist Ronald Munson approaches the point:

> That we don't want a child to be born blind (for example) does not mean we don't value blind people. We value them because they are *people*, though, not because they are blind. People who are blind lack a capacity (sight) that is of value in coping with the world and in appreciating the things in it. The world would be better, in this respect, if those who are blind could see. Yet to say it would be a better world if there were no blind people is not to devalue the people or wish them out of existence. Rather, it is to wish for everyone to possess the capacity of sight.[4]

Now it seems to me that Munson is there giving voice to good common sense. We don't need to value blindness in order to value blind people; and we can value those people while wishing that the condition of blindness did not exist. But can this work as a defence of screening and selective abortion? The trouble is that selective abortion seeks to prevent the condition *by* preventing the lives of those persons who would carry the condition. It cannot attack the condition without attacking the life. There is no *practical* distinction here between the condition, on the one hand, and the individual life in which that condition exists, on the other. Selection seeks to destroy the condition *by* destroying those individual lives.

But now the defenders of selection would respond by claiming that abortion does not involve an attack upon *persons*. Embryonic life and foetal life is not *personal* life, they claim. Foetuses are not persons, for persons emerge *later* in human development. So screening for selective abortion *can* properly be regarded as an attempt to eliminate a *condition*; it does not seek to eliminate persons.

We have arrived, here, at perhaps the most central and disputed issue in the general abortion debate. What significance ought we to attach to unborn human life? What moral status does it possess? Does it have the same moral importance as life after birth, or does it have a lower value – a value that allows us to destroy it under conditions in which we would not be entitled to destroy life after birth? We discussed some arguments addressed to this issue in Chapter Two. There we noted that the embryo or foetus (let us once again simply call it the foetus) is human life. And we might now add that, at least from the time up to which it could twin (which is very early in embryonic development), the foetus is clearly *an individual human life*. We saw in Chapter Two that we would be faced with unacceptable consequences if we claimed that this individual has merely the same significance as a piece of tissue. And we saw that it would be unreasonably arbitrary to claim that birth, or that viability, marks the point where the foetus comes to possess the same moral status as is possessed by a baby; so it must possess that status at an earlier stage. But we saw, too, that our attitude to the natural loss of embryos poses a problem for the view that the foetus has the same moral status as a baby from the moment of its conception. We also mentioned the view that the foetus, though not yet an actual person, is – unlike anything else – a *potential* person. And it seems that *at least* this view must be true, given the fact that the foetus is an individual human life whose natural development is to become a person (if it is not one already). Nevertheless, in noting this fact, we have not yet made its moral implications clear. Ought we so to value potential persons that we treat them with the same care as we treat actual persons? Or are we entitled to attach a lower value to them – and dispose of them under conditions in which we would not be entitled to dispose of actual persons? We have noted these various points and problems, but we have not tried to resolve the issue by fully defining the moral status of the foetus.

And in fact, that issue is only one component of the complicated problem of abortion. In Chapter Two, we heard Judith Jarvis Thomson reminding us that, even if the foetus is to be regarded as a person, the mother has rights and interests which are certainly morally relevant. I argued that Thomson's particular arguments in defence of abortion fail. But she is, of course, quite right to stress that there are two lives involved, and two sets of interests and possible concerns. Those who are in the business of screening for selective abortion are focused primarily on the concerns of the *mother*.

As Rosalind Hursthouse points out, pregnancy is quite unlike any other situation, involving as it does a peculiar and intimate relation between these two lives, and carrying weighty consequences for other lives as well (especially for the father, but also for other family members). The special nature of pregnancy means that a complex range of moral considerations apply to it. And there is a complicated *variety* of ways in which our behaviour in relation to pregnancy might be morally acceptable or otherwise.[5]

Now I shall not attempt to unravel that tangled web here. A proper review of that complicated range of considerations would require its own book-length treatment. But the point to note here is that, because of the complexity of the problem of abortion, the question of the justification of selective abortion of the disabled is not *simply* a question about the value of the lives of the disabled. So if we wish to tackle this latter question, about the value of the lives of the disabled, we cannot do so *straightforwardly* by pursuing the former question, concerning selective abortion.

There is, however, a much more direct way in which to raise the issue of the value of the lives of the disabled. This question is brought into much sharper relief when we consider something advocated by various very influential philosophers for numerous decades. Since the 1970s, the early days of the modern wave of philosophical work in applied ethics, a number of leading philosophers have argued that we are entitled to dispose of the disabled not merely by means of abortion, but by infanticide – by killing disabled babies after they are born.[6] In other words, these philosophers advocate not just selective abortion, but selective infanticide. They are, of course, aware that infanticide is illegal in many jurisdictions; but they are advocating that it is ethically permissible, and that it ought to be legalised.

From selective abortion to selective infanticide

I propose, then, that we examine the case for selective infanticide and compare it with its traditional opposition, for by doing so we will be able to engage much more clearly and directly with the question of the value of the lives of the disabled and our duty of care towards them.

So let us start this examination by imagining a case which raises the ethical issue. A baby has just been born, and it has been born disabled. The disability may be physical, or mental, or both. Now of course, there are many possible disabilities, and much disagreement about how seriously one or other disability compromises the future individual's life. But let's suppose that we agree that this baby's disability is severe. And now we pose the ethical question: what ought we to do with this baby? Ought we to care for it in the way we would care for normal babies? Or are we, indeed, permitted to kill it?

Our ordinary response is to be shocked by the very suggestion that we might kill the baby. In many jurisdictions, this would be murder. And in any case, its prohibition is central to our standard medical ethics. But if we can put our shock aside and cool-headedly consider the question as an ordinary medical issue, we might apply the four principles to the case, arguing as follows. The principle of non-maleficence forbids us to harm the baby by killing it. Rather, we are required by the principle of beneficence to do good to the baby by doing our best to relieve whatever suffering it experiences, and to support it to grow and flourish in whatever ways it can. We cannot now ask the baby what it wishes us to do, as the principle of autonomy would in other cases require. But we can at least attach some sense to the question of what it *would* wish, for we can ask whether it would come to be glad that we had cared for it, rather than killed it. And we can surely offer a well-justified answer to this question, for there are very few disabled adults who claim that they would prefer that we had killed them in their infancy. And in applying the principle of justice, we bring into view a number of further factors. We can claim that the baby possesses the right to life, and that killing it would violate this right. We can claim that fairness demands that we treat this baby as we would treat other babies, and thus that we provide to it the life-supporting care that we standardly provide. But the principle of justice also alerts us to the burden of care that would need to be borne by others (the baby's parents or other carers), and to our duty to do what we fairly and proportionately can to assist these others in bearing that burden. And thus all four principles converge upon the traditional and received view within medical ethics, and the commonly accepted view within the wider community: we ought to preserve the life of this baby, and to support those who are most directly entrusted with its care.[7]

The advocates of infanticide, however, would dispute our application of the four principles. They claim that the baby does not possess a right to life, and that killing it need not be wrong. They claim that we may be doing it harm by extending its life and consequently its suffering, and that the real good we can do to it may be to end its suffering most directly, by killing it. They claim that the principle of autonomy simply does not apply to babies, so it falls away as irrelevant. And they claim that the interests of third parties – given the burden of care that would fall upon others, and the fact (when it is a fact) that the parents do not want this baby – may themselves be sufficient to justify the killing of the baby.

Thus, in offering positive grounds for infanticide, the advocates are appealing to the two factors which they regard as relevant – the baby's future suffering, and the burden caused to others by the baby's continued existence and need for care. They argue that either of these factors, or the combination of them, could entail that the best outcome would be the death of the baby, and that in that case we ought to be able to bring about its death most directly – by killing it.

It cannot be denied, I think, that the advocates of infanticide are there appealing to factors which ought to concern us all. In the previous chapter, we noted that a limit to our duty to prolong life occurs at the point where in doing so, we are imposing on the patient a burden which is too much to bear. Some babies are born with incurable conditions which cause relentless and extreme suffering, and in such cases we must hope that their pain and distress can be well managed and that their lives will not be unduly extended. But thankfully, most disabilities (including most disabilities for which pre-natal screening is done) are not as extreme as that. Nevertheless, many of these conditions will certainly involve suffering, and we should indeed be concerned both about the future suffering of the disabled baby and about the burden upon others of its care. And if we can put aside our worry about violating the traditional prohibition of killing, we can feel the inclination to think along the lines opened out by the advocates of infanticide. "Taking everything into account, wouldn't it be better if this life were to end now?" we might ask. "But if that's so, oughtn't we to be allowed to *bring* this life to an end now?"

There is some common ground, then, between the traditional, generally accepted view that we should preserve and care for the newborn life, on the one hand, and the advocacy of infanticide, on the other. And yet there is a yawning chasm between those two positions. Let us probe further to see what gives rise to this great difference. The central difference arises because the advocates of infanticide reject the related notions of the prohibition against killing, the right to life of the baby, and so on. The contrast between the views is often very simply expressed by pointing out that they disagree concerning a central idea or doctrine that has exerted a powerful influence in our thinking about such issues – the doctrine of the sanctity of human life. What is this doctrine?

The sanctity of human life

There are a number of possible versions of the idea of the sanctity of life. In much ethical discussion, this doctrine is taken to say simply that human life is intrinsically valuable, valuable in itself; or that taking human life is intrinsically wrong. Those who actually hold the doctrine in this way believe that there is something wrong with killing (of humans) *as such*. They may not believe that it is *always* wrong, or that it is overridingly wrong: they may believe that it can be justified in special circumstances (e.g., in self-defence, or war, or perhaps in capital punishment). But they believe that when those special circumstances do *not* obtain, we do not need to look for some particular reason why it would be wrong to destroy human life. Rather, they believe, we can recognise that it would be wrong *just because* it would be a killing of someone; it would be *intrinsically* wrong, or wrong in itself. This, as I say, is what many contemporary philosophers and ethicists *mean* by the doctrine of the sanctity of life. Some of them accept the doctrine, so interpreted, and some of them don't.

But there is also a more substantial reading of the doctrine. The word "sanctity" has what some people would call "religious" connotations. In its proper sense, it applies to what is set apart as holy and for that reason to be revered, or to be regarded as inviolable, or especially to be protected, and so on. And it is not difficult to see why someone who accepts this richer notion of the sanctity of human life would also accept the simpler notion that the philosophers work with. For ease of reference, I will call that simpler notion the "thinner" doctrine of the sanctity of life, and the richer, more "religious" notion the "thicker" doctrine.

So the contrast between the two opposing positions concerning infanticide can be described in very simple terms as a disagreement over the thinner doctrine of the sanctity of life. The traditional, common view holds that it is intrinsically wrong to destroy human life (and thus the life of the baby); whereas the advocates of infanticide believe that this doctrine is false, and that our ethics should be constructed according to an alternative view concerning the significance of life and of its destruction.

But then, what should we say about this doctrine of the sanctity of human life? What reason can be offered for it?

Many of us incline to the doctrine simply because we feel intuitively that it is correct. We have a deep sense that the killing of a human being would be wrong in itself. We feel that, in fundamental respects, the life of the disabled baby is as important, as morally significant, as the life of a normal (or non-disabled) baby; just as we feel that the life of a disabled adult is as important as the life of a normal adult. We feel that the killing of the disabled baby would be, in fundamental respects, as serious as the killing of a normal baby, just as we feel that the killing of a disabled adult would be as serious as the killing of a non-disabled adult. We feel that each killing would be seriously wrong – just because it is a killing of a human being. We may express this by saying that there is a moral prohibition against killing which applies equally to all humans, whether disabled or otherwise. We may well wish to say that each of these humans possesses the right to life. And when we are pressed to say why we believe these things, we may be able to answer only that they are deep moral intuitions of ours. After all, *any* moral outlook must have at its foundation basic intuitions, and these are some of ours.

That is a perfectly possible position. In the earlier chapters, we have repeatedly noted the importance of our moral intuitions, which emerge from our moral sense. Unless we have such a sense, we cannot perform what is truly *our own* moral appreciation or evaluation of anything. And some of the intuitions which emerge from our moral sense must stand at the foundations of our moral outlook. They will be intuitions which provide the *basis* for our other moral beliefs, and thus intuitions which have no further basis themselves.

Nevertheless, concerning the sanctity of life, many of us will be inclined to say more. For many accept the thinner doctrine because they accept the thicker doctrine too. The thicker doctrine provides a ground for the thinner one. We see the thicker doctrine emerge clearly from the theistic world-view which we reviewed in Chapter Three. According to this view, human life is set apart under a special protective commandment of God. We are commanded not to kill other human beings; indeed, we are commanded to love them. Humans, on this picture, were created in God's image. And however broken and spoiled we are now, we remain loved by God, who is, at his own cost, in the business of seeking to redeem us and transform us into the kinds of persons he intends that we should be forever. On this picture, each human being is damaged, and thus we are *all*, to some extent, *disabled*. None of us is *truly* normal. But each of us has a unique and incalculable value – a value that is due to our relation to God and God's purposes. The term "alien dignity" is sometimes used to describe this significance of the human individual. Each of us possesses a value, a significance, which is not due to our own intrinsic natural qualities, but is bestowed upon us by *another* – by God, in his love for us. So the value of each human life is not a function of our natural abilities, or the condition of our bodies, or our usefulness, or the extent to which we are wanted by other humans, or any other aspect of our natural life: it is a function of God's love and transcendent purposes for us.

It is very interesting to note that this picture gave rise to the outlook and inspiration of many of those who established our hospitals or made other provision for individuals at the margins of human life – for the disabled, the weak, the vulnerable, the poor, the disturbed, the deranged, the dispossessed, the unwanted. And our more recent public institutions have been modelled on those earlier provisions of care. The founders of those services frequently appealed to this notion of the transcendent, alien dignity of each human individual. It was what moved them to extend care to all, however compromised the life of those they served. The same motivation animates the work of the countless different people and organisations around the world who persist in these provisions of care. If we wished to have before our minds a prominent recent example of this outlook in action, we could think of Mother Teresa. She, of course, was the famous Roman Catholic nun who founded the Missionaries of Charity, whose work – in India and elsewhere – was devoted to the care of the poorest of the poor. She claimed to see each compromised human life as the life of someone loved by God and bearing a dignity bestowed by God. And in particular, she insisted that we are required to provide to disabled babies just as much life-supporting care as we would provide to normal babies. She and her community famously *extended* that care to such babies, embracing them in love and providing homes and support for those that had been abandoned. And she strongly opposed the view that these lives, or any human lives, are to be neglected, and even more strongly opposed the view that they may be destroyed.[8]

But the advocates of infanticide reject that theistic picture, and they also reject the thinner doctrine of the sanctity of life. What, then, is their alternative picture of the significance of life and death? We need to spend a little while in examining this, and for that purpose I shall concentrate upon the early landmark account offered by the English philosopher Jonathan Glover.[9] (The account proposed later by the Australian philosopher Peter Singer is substantially the same as Glover's.)[10] Glover's (and Singer's) approach is broadly utilitarian. Now we saw, in Chapter Four, powerful reasons to reject utilitarianism. Does this mean that we can reject Glover's account of the ethics of life and death? No. That would, at least at this stage, be an unjustified conclusion. As we saw in Chapter Two, a false view or theory can nevertheless have true consequences. (To suppose otherwise is to commit the fallacy of denying the antecedent.) Perhaps Glover has arguments which show us that we should abandon the doctrine of the sanctity of life and embrace instead his alternative account. So let us examine his arguments.

Jonathan Glover's arguments for infanticide

As we saw in Chapter Four, the utilitarian will evaluate a killing, or the supporting of a life, in terms of its *consequences*. So it follows immediately, according to the utilitarian, that no killing of a human being is wrong just because it is a killing of a human being. It will be wrong – or right, as the case may be – because of its consequences. And to evaluate the killing, the moral question we need to ask is whether it maximises the good. For our moral duty is to bring about the greatest total of good (once the consequent bad has been subtracted from the consequent good). And what is the good? We saw that different utilitarians give slightly different answers to that question, but that the classical utilitarian's answer is that the good is happiness (and the bad is suffering). Glover's answer to the question is rather less simple than the classical utilitarian's answer, for he is not sure that everything that we should count as good can be clearly connected with happiness. He refers instead to those things which contribute to a life worth living, but he does not try to provide a list of what those things are. So he would say that our moral duty is to bring about the greatest net total of those things that make life worth living. But in discussing this, I will sometimes simply use the term "happiness" to include whatever might be included among those things which make life worth living, as Glover would want them to be included.

How does Glover apply this to our question about what to do with the baby? He points out that there are two sets of consequences that we must consider. *First*, we must consider those matters that *directly* concern the baby's life. How much good would the baby's future life contain? Would that future individual's life contain more happiness (or more of those things that make life worth living) than suffering, or *vice versa*? We are asking here whether the infant has before it a worthwhile life – a life preferable to death. Glover points out that it can be very difficult to imagine this future life, and therefore difficult to answer this question, and that different people may well give different answers. But he says that the best way to answer it will be "for us to ask whether we ourselves would find such a life preferable to death".[11] And if our answer is that we would opt for death rather than that life, then we have an argument for killing the baby now.

The *second* set of consequences we need to consider, according to Glover, are the *indirect* consequences of killing the baby or keeping it alive – that is, the consequences in the lives of *other* people. Glover calls these consequences *side-effects*. So here we need to consider whether the baby's life would lead to more suffering than happiness for the other people involved (the family, friends, medical team, and so on), or *vice versa*. In particular, we need to consider what the parents want. "The parents ... are likely to be greatly distressed by the killing of their baby," Glover points out. "But ... this may be less terrible for the parents than having to live with their child and bring him up. It is an unpalatable truth that appeals to side-effects can sometimes be among the strongest arguments *for* infanticide."[12]

In his general discussion of the ethics of killing, Glover introduces a *third* consideration: he believes that when we are considering whether someone's life ought to go on, we should also consider whether that persons *wants* to go on living. In other words, we ought to respect that person's *autonomy*. This is not a strictly utilitarian consideration because it does not concern the consequences of the action. Nevertheless, Glover believes that it is a factor – though not an overriding factor – which needs to be taken into account along with the other relevant considerations. However, he points out that babies cannot understand the choice between death and life: they simply do not possess the concepts one would need to possess in order to be able to grasp that distinction. So they cannot have a preference here one way or the other, and so the question of respect for their autonomy cannot arise. And so, he says, this consideration falls out of the picture when we are discussing infanticide.

Thus, our question about what to do with the baby is, according to Glover, to be answered by considering, first, the direct consequences, and secondly, the indirect consequences of killing the baby, on the one hand, and of keeping the baby alive, on the other. Of course, it may be a very difficult and complicated matter to predict and evaluate those two kinds of consequences. It may be that the baby's future life would contain a complex mixture of happiness and suffering. It may be that the side-effects of taking that life would also involve both happiness and suffering. We also need to consider the longer-term social consequences of a *policy* of permitting infanticide. And so on. But if we can reasonably predict that the greatest good is to be obtained by taking the baby's life, then it will be permissible, and could even be obligatory, to kill the baby.

We see, then, how Glover's way of tackling the issue embraces the two concerns which we all share – the quality of the baby's future life, and the burden of care imposed upon others. But for Glover, those concerns are nested among a wider series of claims, and there are many points at which his claims can be challenged. To start with, is he right to dismiss autonomy from the list of applicable considerations? At the beginning of our discussion of the baby's case, I suggested a way in which we can see that autonomy is in fact relevant. Let's agree with Glover that infants are now conceptually unable to entertain a preference concerning ongoing life or death. But is there nevertheless not a sense in which we can ask what they *would* prefer? Consider a man in a coma who has a real prospect of recovery of consciousness. He is unable now to entertain any preference, so we cannot sensibly ask whether he *does* now prefer to go on living or to die. But we can sensibly ask what he *would* prefer; and we can work towards an actual answer to that question by asking whether, if we now kept him alive, he would be disappointed or grateful, once he had regained consciousness, that we had kept him alive. And by considering his future prospects, we may have very good grounds for a reasonable answer to that question. Indeed, this is surely a question that we *should* be ready to ask. But now, isn't that case parallel in relevant respects to the case of an infant? We can ask, and surely we should ask, whether the future individual would be grateful that we had kept him or her alive. So isn't Glover wrong to hold that the question of respect for autonomy simply does not arise in the case of an infant? And when we do ask what this individual *would* prefer, aren't we often able to give a very positive answer to the question? As I mentioned earlier, there are very few disabled adults who would prefer that they had been killed as infants. (We need to be careful, of course, to ask the correct question here. It is not "Would this individual prefer not to be disabled?", for that does not refer to an option that we can bring about. The question is rather "Would this individual prefer no life at all rather than this life as a disabled person?")[13]

And there can be various ways in which we are worried by Glover's question concerning the value of the baby's future life. For instance, we might object to Glover's claim that *we ourselves* ought to evaluate whether this individual's future life would be worthwhile. We might well feel that we have *no right* to make such an assessment. And we could certainly feel that we lack the *competence* to do so. Glover himself points out that this assessment can require a very difficult exercise of imagination. (*What would it be like* to live with this particular disability?) But in any case, if the question must be raised, isn't there in fact a much more reliable way to approach it? Why shouldn't we answer it not by appealing to what we imagine our own preferences would be, but by finding out the preferences of people who actually experience that kind of life? Many of those people would be able to tell us whether they would prefer to go on living or to die. They would be able to indicate that their life is so bad that they would prefer to have been killed as infants, if that were indeed the case. (Yet they typically do *not* tell us that.) And even when their disability is so serious that they cannot give us a coherent statement that they wish to go on living, we may still be able to discern that we would do them no service by ending their life.

However, we might well be disturbed by the *very asking* of that question. We may feel, as I mentioned, that we have no right to ask whether someone else's life is worthwhile, because we feel that we have no right to act – in effect – as judge of whether they should live or die. For this is, after all, why Glover insists that we ask the question: we do so in order to determine that individual's fate. Furthermore, we can be very properly disturbed, it seems to me, when we consider what our asking of this question implies for those people who live with the sorts of disabilities we are evaluating. We noted earlier that our very discussion of screening and selective abortion can be felt as offensive, and indeed threatening, to people who live with disability; and this must be even more true of our discussion of infanticide. Whenever we decide that life with such a disability would not be worthwhile, and that we would therefore be entitled to kill the baby, we are in effect saying to someone who lives with that disability, "*Your* life is not worthwhile and we would have been justified in killing *you* when you were an infant."

Still, those challenges notwithstanding, many people – certainly many philosophers – endorse Glover's approach to the issue. And many welcome the fact that by thinking about life and death along these lines, we are thinking in what seem to be reasonable terms. We are thinking about it by considering the good and the bad that are evident in the real, natural world – the good and the bad that we can get some real grip upon, and weigh up and rationally assess. We are thinking about it, in particular, without having to be encumbered by unwelcome vestiges of an old but now unlamented "religious" tradition.

But I think that it is particularly revealing to probe Glover's picture yet further and carefully examine its consequences. Glover has replaced the doctrine of the sanctity of life with his own account of the value of life. What is good about life? What value does it have? Simply put, the heart of his answer is that the value of life consists in what it *contains*. Life is not valuable in itself: its value consists in its containing those things that make life worth living. *Those things* are the good, not life itself. The value of life is its value only as a *container*; it is what the container *contains* that matters. But this means that the container doesn't matter *at all* so long as the value of what it contains can be preserved. Indeed, it doesn't matter if the container gets destroyed so long as you don't lose the value of the contents. Peter Singer (whose view of life and death is broadly the same as Glover's) puts it like this. It is, he says, as if "sentient beings are receptacles of something valuable and it does not matter if a receptacle gets broken, so long as there is another receptacle to which the contents can be transferred without any getting spilt".[14]

And as Glover points out, this means that babies are *replaceable*. As he puts it:

> ... newborn babies ... are replaceable. It is wrong to kill a baby who has a good chance of having a worth-while life, but ... it would not be wrong to kill him if the alternative to his existence was the existence of someone else with an equally good chance of a life at least as worth-while.[15]

And to illustrate his point, he goes on to say this:

> If a mother is resolved to have exactly one child and no more, the death of her first baby may cause her to have another. If the second baby has just as good a life as the first one would have done, then ... the death of the first baby has not mattered at all.[16]

What Glover is saying here emerges quite clearly from his ethical framework, and its significance needs to be taken very seriously. He is not just talking about disabled babies here; he is talking about *all babies*, including perfectly healthy babies. He is saying that it is all right to kill a baby so long as we can replace it with another one with an equally worthwhile future life. The baby's life, the baby itself, is just the container for future good. The container can be destroyed so long as we can keep the same amount of good contents. If we do kill the first baby and replace it with an equally promising second baby, then "the death of the first baby has not mattered at all".

Now, I invite us to consider whether this is acceptable. Do we agree that in the imagined situation the death of the first baby *has not mattered at all*?

Many of us are shocked by this suggestion. (Certainly my students are shocked. For I regularly put this question to them, and watch their reactions.) We feel that the death of the first baby certainly does matter. And thus we feel that we see here an unacceptable consequence of Glover's view.

However, I must confess that I haven't yet been quite fair to Glover. For what he says here is qualified, and I have omitted that qualification until now. The relevant sentences, which include Glover's qualification, are as follows:

> It is wrong to kill a baby who has a good chance of having a worth-while life, but *in terms of this objection* it would not be wrong to kill him if the alternative to his existence was the existence of someone else with an equally good chance of a life at least as worth-while.[17]

And: "If the second baby has just as good a life as the first one would have done, then, in terms of the worth-while life objection, the death of the first baby has not mattered at all."[18]

What does this qualification ("in terms of this objection") mean? Glover is concerned here only with the *direct* consequences of killing – consequences involving those matters "that relate solely to the person killed"[19]. And those matters are the amounts of happiness and suffering within this life. So, if you can kill the baby painlessly, and replace it with another equally promising baby, then *as far as the direct consequences are concerned*, the death of the first baby does not matter at all, for you retain the same amount of good as would have been contained within the life of the first baby. But Glover is not saying that the baby's death does not matter in *any* way. For in addition to direct consequences, there are indirect consequences or side-effects – the consequences for *other* people. And the first baby's death might have bad consequences for other people, and so it might matter in *that* way. Indeed, Glover thinks that the side-effects of infanticide are what can justify our reluctance to accept that it is all right to kill babies and replace them.

Now, of course, the killing of a baby is likely to have real side-effects: the parents might suffer grief or at least self-reproach (even if the baby is being killed because they don't want it); the killing could be messy and disgusting; it might cause distress for the medical team appointed to do the killing; and so on. But do these factors provide a *complete* explanation of how the death of the first baby *could* matter? Again, I invite us to consider that question.

Many of us (including my students) are unimpressed. We reject the suggestion that these factors provide the *only* reason why the death of the first baby matters. And as we think about this question, it is not hard to find arguments for saying that this appeal to side-effects cannot be a complete explanation.

First, we can perform a little thought experiment. We can imagine a situation in which a perfectly healthy and normal baby is killed and replaced *without* there being any bad side-effects. Suppose, for instance, that the baby's parents will suffer no grief or discomfort because they don't want the baby and really do want it to die. (Perhaps they want a boy rather than this girl. Perhaps they want a baby not *now* but later...) And suppose that the killing is carried out by a well-trained clinical team of utilitarians who have got over any misplaced feelings of distress, and who can perform the killing cleanly and efficiently. And suppose that the killing is done secretly so that other people aren't distressed or caused to fear the clinical team. And so on. (As usual, to frame the required hypothetical situation, we need only let our imaginations run in relevant directions.) Now we have eliminated bad side-effects of the killing. And as we think about our imagined situation, where the first baby is killed and later replaced by a second one, would it *now* be true to say that the death of the first baby *does not matter at all* – that it does not matter morally, that nothing morally wrong or even morally questionable occurs? Again, many of us reject this suggestion. We still think that the death of the first baby matters, precisely because it is the destruction of an individual. We may well feel that the right descriptive word is still "murder", which still carries all the moral weight that it normally carries. Indeed, many people think that what we are contemplating here is *worse* than what would standardly be described as murder, for they feel that there is something *especially* wrong about the killing of a baby. And the fact that the baby is replaced is irrelevant to this evaluation.

That, then, is the first argument. Here is a second one. We can point out that Glover's appeal to side-effects seems to reverse the proper order of the logic of the matter. It's not that the killing of the baby is a bad thing *because* the parents will grieve or the medical team will be distressed. It's that the parents will grieve and the medical team will be distressed because the killing is a bad thing! The morally important side-effects are due to the badness of the killing, not the other way around.

So Glover fails to convince at least many of us that killing the baby and replacing it matters, if it matters at all, only because of the side-effects of the killing. We find this to be an untenable consequence of this theory.

But it is not the only such consequence. In his discussion, he points out that the fact that the baby would have a worthwhile future life would count as an objection to the killing of the baby. And we have seen what he means by this. He means, of course, that if you killed such a baby, you would be lessening the amount of good in the world; and therefore, unless it were replaced (and leaving aside side-effects), its killing would be wrong. But then he goes on to say that this is a "relatively weak" objection.[20] Why is it a weak objection to the killing of the baby? For the following reason: "even where the worth-while life argument does hold, it is no stronger against infanticide than against not conceiving a child. In either case, there is one less person with a worth-while life."[21]

What is Glover saying here? He is noting that on his theory it is wrong, other things being equal, to prevent the good in the baby's future worthwhile life. But he is pointing out that – apart from killing – there is also another way of preventing that future good. You would prevent that future good by not conceiving the baby in the first place – by refraining from sexual activity, or by using contraception. So, as far as this consideration is concerned, infanticide, on the one hand, and not conceiving a child, on the other, are *morally on a par*. And this means that if it is very wrong to kill a baby, then it is just as wrong not to conceive a baby. Alternatively, if it is morally acceptable not to conceive a baby, then it is just as morally acceptable to kill a baby. (We are assuming that the babies we are talking about can be expected to have a similarly worthwhile life. And we are leaving side-effects out of the picture.)

Is this an acceptable consequence of Glover's theory? I now invite us to consider this question. Glover draws this consequence to our attention precisely in order to persuade us that we should be willing to accept that infanticide is permissible. If we accept that it is all right not to conceive a child then – so the argument goes – we should similarly accept that it is all right to kill the baby. But once again, many of us are entirely unconvinced. *Of course* killing a baby is morally very different to not conceiving a baby, we very naturally say. Not conceiving a baby is one thing, morally speaking. Killing a baby is quite another. There is no moral comparison: killing a baby is very much worse!

This natural intuitive reaction seems, as we reflect upon it, to be quite right. There is surely an important moral difference between killing and not-conceiving. In the one case – killing – there is an individual human being who is destroyed. Nothing like that, morally speaking, is happening in the case of not-conceiving – in the not-conceiving of any one of the countless merely possible babies that any of us could conceive. Imagine, for instance, a large number of men and women who all happen to be fertile at the moment and all happen to be within striking distance of one another (perhaps within one building), but who are all going about their own ordinary business and not engaging in any sexual activity while doing so. Take one particular man and one particular woman in that group. It is true that this man *could* generate a child with this woman now, or with this woman not now, but a minute later, or two minutes later, or an hour later, and so on. It is also true that this man could generate a child not with *this* woman, but with one of the *other* women now, or a minute later, and so on. And it is true that a *different* particular man could generate a child with this woman now, or a different woman now, or later, and so on and so on. But none of them is doing this. These are all instances of not-conceiving, and we see that there is an enormous – a genuinely indefinite – number of them. And so there is an indefinite number of possible babies that are not being conceived by the men and women in that group. Those men and women are deliberately doing other things; they are in the business of *not* conceiving any of those possible babies. (And if it occurs to them that they *could* be conceiving one or other of those possible babies, then they are deliberately *choosing* not to do so.) And what is true of those men and women is true of most of us most of the time. We are in the business of not-conceiving babies nearly all the time. And Glover wants us to believe that *each time* we don't conceive a baby, we are doing something morally on a par with *killing a baby* (apart from side-effects). What he wants us to believe, therefore, means one of two possible things. Either we are, nearly all the time, while going about our ordinary business, repeatedly doing something as morally serious as killing a baby. And that surely cannot be correct. Or killing a baby is no more morally serious than any of the ordinary things we do most of the time. And that cannot be correct either. The not-conceiving of one of the indefinite number of possible babies we *could* conceive is of a different order to the killing of the actual baby. The cases are not morally on a par.

But Glover might reply. He might repeat that killing and not-conceiving are morally on a par insofar as they prevent future good. And there are many ways, he can point out, of bringing about future good: conceiving a worthwhile life is just one of those ways. So if the people who are choosing not to conceive babies are, while going about their ordinary business, bringing about good in *other* ways, then their activity is *not* morally on a par with killing babies. They could, indeed, be doing things which are as morally significant as conceiving children. (Whereas if they are not bringing about significant good in other ways, then their not-conceiving could indeed be morally on a par with killing.) So, in appealing to the fact that we are engaged in countless not-conceivings, I have failed to show that killing and not-conceiving are not on a par.

Is this a successful reply? It might pacify us if we supposed that everything we ordinarily do is morally valuable – on a par with bringing a worthwhile life into the world. But we do not suppose this. Consider again our various possible pairs of men and women in the group we imagined earlier who are choosing not to conceive a child. Suppose that they choose, instead, to chat about the weather, or to have coffee together, or to ignore one another while dealing with their respective email messages. Are we to say that in choosing these things, they are doing something as morally significant as bringing a worthwhile life into the world? Surely not. But are we therefore to say that what they are doing is morally on a par with killing a baby? Again, surely not.

But Glover can also reply by appealing to side-effects (as he did when he sought to convince us that the killing of a baby does not matter at all, so long as it is replaced). For, of course, he would be right to point out that conceiving a child certainly does have consequences for persons other than the child. But can this provide a *complete* explanation of why not-conceiving can be morally different from killing? If our possible pairs of men and women within that group are to choose to conceive a child, they need to experience intimate activity together.

For some of them, no doubt, this will be an unwelcome prospect. But surely not for all. Many people testify that the process is rather pleasant. Then, of course, there are serious consequences for the mother: she has to endure a pregnancy which can be burdensome, and a labour which can be painful and dangerous. Well, let us tinker with our thought experiment and imagine that all the females in the group are among those lucky women who find pregnancy on the whole unburdensome and labour easy. And let us suppose that in the background there is a plentiful supply of possible foster parents who would be happy to assume the care of consequent babies, and perhaps ready to pay the mother something for her trouble. And let us suppose that the women and their possible male partners nevertheless persist in going about their ordinary business, choosing *not* to conceive children together. Are we *now* to say that in doing this they are doing what is morally the same as *killing babies*? Again, surely not. We have removed bad side-effects from our imagined situation, but we still do not have a moral equivalence between killing and not-conceiving. Side-effects cannot supply a complete explanation of the difference between them.

Thus we have identified what certainly seem to very many of us to be two unacceptable consequences of Glover's way of thinking about life and death. On Glover's theory, if a baby is killed and replaced by another equally promising baby, then (apart from side-effects) the death of the first baby has not mattered at all. And secondly, killing a baby is (apart from side-effects) no worse than not conceiving a baby. Glover draws our attention to these consequences in order to try to help us to accept his theory and his argument that infanticide is permissible. But those of us who regard these consequences as unacceptable will take exactly the opposite course. We will reject his theory. For as we know, if a theory has any false consequence, then the theory is false.

And if we are indeed right to say that those consequences of Glover's theory are unacceptable, then something very interesting seems to follow immediately concerning the value of human life. Why is it that when a baby is killed but replaced its death does matter? Why is it that parents grieve the loss of a baby, even when they go on to have another baby with an equally good life? Because they have lost *that individual human being*. They have lost not a mere "it", but that little child, whom they could name, and whose name was its own, not anyone else's. That unique individual has been lost, and *cannot be replaced*. The parents can have *other* children, but they cannot replace *that* child, who possessed *his or her own unique value*. Indeed, the parents may feel that Glover's talk of replacement here is an obscene misuse of the word – that it is offensive even to suggest that their precious child can be replaced.

But note what follows. If the individual's loss does matter, even though we can retain the amount of good that would have been contained within his or her life, then this individual life itself matters. This life itself has value. If the destruction of an individual life matters more than the not-conceiving of any one of the uncountably many merely possible babies that one could conceive, this is again because it is the destruction of an actual individual, with his or her own unique value. The individual life matters in itself. It has its own value, regardless of what it can contain. We seem, then, to have arrived back squarely at the thinner doctrine of the sanctity of human life, simply by observing where Glover's theory leads us astray.

Back to the sanctity of human life

Now, in drawing these conclusions – in arriving back at the sanctity of life in this way – we are of course relying on our own moral sense, our moral intuitions. But – to stress the point again – there is nothing wrong with our doing this. Philosophers – including Glover – all test their theories against their own and other people's moral intuitions. If we had no moral sense of our own upon which we could rely, then we would have nothing against which we could assess the basic assumptions of any moral theory. Glover and others are, of course, proposing their moral theory on the alleged ground that its basic tenets square with what our moral sense tells us. We are all appealing to the deliverances of our own moral sense.

In response to our arguments against him, Glover will have no objection to our appeal to intuitions. And he certainly won't dispute the validity of our reasoning. He agrees that those are consequences of his theory. Indeed, he drew them to our attention. And he agrees that if those consequences are false, then his theory is false. But he disagrees that those consequences are false. He accepts them. He believes his theory, so he embraces those consequences. (His case is an argument in the form of modus ponens.) We believe that those consequences are unacceptable, so we reject his theory. (Our case is an argument in the form of modus tollens.) And in our rejection of the consequences of his theory, we appear to have accepted once again the thinner doctrine of the sanctity of life. That is the state of play in the discussion so far.

All the same, I still have not been entirely fair to Glover. For he has further argument for his theory – or at least for that part of his theory which denies the sanctity of life. He invites us to join him in some thought experiments in order to test the idea that life is valuable not just because of the good things it can contain, but in itself.[22] The first thought experiment is this: imagine two different situations – one where you have died (and ceased to exist); the other in which you remain in a *permanent* coma. The only difference between those situations is, of course, that in one of them you are alive, and in the other you are not. Now, Glover asks, is there any reason to prefer the permanent coma to death? No there's not, he feels. And this shows that there is no value to be attached to *mere* life; to life in itself. Suppose, then, that someone responds to this argument by claiming that it is not mere life which is valuable in itself, but *conscious* life. Well, says Glover, now perform a revised thought experiment. Consider a different pair of situations. The first, once again, is a situation in which you have died. The second is a situation in which you are conscious, but *merely* conscious – nothing else. You have no emotional responses to anything, and you *can't take an interest* in anything. As Glover puts it, the conscious being in this situation "cannot be pleased or sorry or in pain; it cannot be interested or bored; it is merely aware of its environment".[23] Glover feels that there is no reason to prefer this second situation to the first. So he concludes that there is nothing intrinsically valuable about merely conscious life. And so he rejects the doctrine of the sanctity of life. He concludes that life, even conscious life, is valuable not in itself, but only because of what it can contain.

Now I think that we could wrestle with those thought experiments for some time. But the point I want to make here is that they do *not* provide for Glover a decisive argument against the doctrine of the sanctity of life. I think that his thought experiments do cause us to wonder about the value of *genuinely bare, genuinely empty* life. But this doesn't show that human life doesn't have a value more fundamental than, and not dependent upon, what it naturally contains. For instance, it doesn't show that the thicker doctrine of the sanctity of life is false. On the theistic picture we have noted earlier, each individual human life has its own incalculable value – however broken and degraded and empty it may now be as far as its natural qualities are concerned. It is true that, strictly speaking, life is not, on that picture, *intrinsically* valuable, for its value is due to its relation to God – to God's purposes for it, and God's valuation of it. But its value is not dependent on what Glover believes give life its only value – the worthwhile things that it naturally contains now. Its value transcends the natural.

A limited little analogy may help. Suppose that a particularly precious diamond, one of the crown jewels, gets lost. And suppose that I stumble upon it. I happen to know nothing of the crown jewels. I know nothing even of diamonds. I pick up this object, and I look at it. I may quite like the look of it. But once I have grown tired of looking at it and carting it around, and seeing no other value in it, I am inclined to throw it away. Is my valuation of it correct? Am I acting in a way that is consistent with its real value? Of course not. I cannot just by looking at this object appreciate its real value. Simply by looking at it, I cannot see that it has been acquired at enormous cost; that it would be recovered at enormous cost; that it has been fashioned in order to take its part within a beautifully designed, splendid and immensely precious collection. Its enormous value transcends what I, in my ignorance, can see.

It seems to me that Glover's thought experiments are as reliable a test of the value of life as my ignorant consideration of the diamond is a reliable valuation of the diamond. So I am not persuaded by his further arguments for his theory, insofar as it entails the denial of the sanctity of life. And, along with many others, I remain convinced that we have identified unacceptable consequences of his theory (which therefore show that his theory is false).

Peter Singer regards the doctrine of the sanctity of human life as *speciesist* – as a mere self-serving prejudice, an unwarranted preference for our own species over others (as racism is an unwarranted favouring of one's own race, or as sexism of one's own sex). But the special valuing of human life is not unwarranted if the thicker doctrine is true. For on the theistic picture, human life has a distinct value and purpose in God's scheme of things, and it is placed under his special protection. We are prohibited from destroying human life except when there is special moral justification for doing so. It should also be pointed out that the biblical theistic picture provides no genuine ground for the abuse of non-human life. However that picture might have been misapplied, it in fact stipulates that humans are to exercise a caring stewardship over the whole of God's world, and we cannot perform that role properly unless we pay due regard to the interests of all creatures. It should be a matter of common sense that we have a duty not to impose unwarranted suffering on sentient animals – the animals which can feel.

In fact, Singer understands very clearly how the thinner doctrine can be related to the thicker one, for he takes pains to *blame* the theistic picture for the thinner doctrine, which he rejects. He stresses that the doctrine of the sanctity of life was introduced into the world by Christianity.[24] He wants us to understand that infanticide was common, indeed sometimes obligatory, in the Graeco-Roman world and in many other cultures. Historians inform me that he is right about this. And Singer wants this fact to help us to embrace infanticide. He regards this as a reason why we can forget our qualms about killing disabled babies: we can give up our opposition to infanticide because we have given up our adherence to Christianity. That, as we have seen, is one direction in which the reasoning can travel. But if we feel that we are right in our rejection of the consequences of Glover's and Singer's theory, we will not reason in that direction. Instead, we may well be grateful for the fact that Christianity has endorsed what our intuitions suggest is true – and thankful that it has thereby afforded protection to countless babies who would otherwise have perished, just as we can be thankful for the fact that it moved cultures to give up human sacrifice, and the glorification of suicide, and slavery, and enjoyment in watching people slaughter one another in the arena. We can be grateful, in other words, for those ways in which Christianity moved those societies to recognise and protect the value of lives which had been regarded as disposable. We can be grateful, too, that Christianity moved people to establish hospitals and to care for the sick – to care for human life however damaged, or diseased, or deranged, or weak, or helpless. We can be grateful that it moved people to set up various other compassionate, charitable organisations, extending care to orphans, to the aged, to the unwanted, and to others in need. And we can be grateful for the fact that it provided a comfortable intellectual home for a whole cluster of human rights. We can be immensely grateful that the Christian picture not only persuaded people of the truth of the value of human life, however compromised that life, but also *moved* those people *to act* as they believed.

Does this mean that the thicker doctrine is correct? Have we just been presented with reason to regard the theistic picture as true? We need to be careful here. The theistic picture does endorse the intuitions to which I have been appealing. It is one of the *consequences* of that picture that each human life possesses its own unique value. But this is not enough to justify our concluding that the theistic picture is true. For as we know, false theories can have consequences which happen to be true. (We must be careful to avoid the fallacy of affirming the consequent.) The theistic picture may not be the only possible theory that can account for the thinner version of the doctrine of the sanctity of life.

Nevertheless, it might perhaps be the case that the theistic picture provides the *best explanation* of the sanctity of human life. That is an interesting possibility. In order to examine it, let's marshal the relevant facts, recalling what we noted in Chapter Two about how an inference to the best explanation works.

What are the data that we would be seeking to explain here? There is the fact that we (or at least many of us) possess a powerful *intuition* that each human life, however damaged, has its own special value and deserves to be protected and cared for. And there is the fact that people such as Mother Teresa have been *motivated* to extend that care to lives that would otherwise have been abandoned or disposed of. But there is also another, related phenomenon needing to be explained. When we witness the work of Mother Teresa, or the countless others who care for damaged or unwanted human lives, many of us find ourselves *inspired* by what we see. We may well be embarrassed by the contrast between our own behaviour and the work of those carers, but we are nevertheless inspired by the very remarkable *love* there on display.[25]

Now Glover and Singer and others would claim that these data can be eliminated. The intuition is false, and should be expunged. And the inspiration is misplaced. For the love shown by Mother Teresa and the others is in fact misguided. In extending that committed, life-supporting care to those damaged or unwanted humans, the carers are in fact perpetuating life which may not be worthwhile, and which can, and perhaps should, be destroyed and replaced. So

Glover and Singer would claim. But many of us find these claims unconvincing – not to mention thoroughly objectionable. We feel that our intuition is in fact a reliable guide to the truth. And we feel that the inspiration we receive is very proper: we feel that the carers are demonstrating a love which is deeply admirable, and that our being inspired by it is a *fitting* response to what we observe.

Those, then, are the data needing to be explained. And what is the hypothesis being considered as the best explanation? That, of course, is the theistic picture which we described in Chapter Three.

Now in Chapter Two, we saw how it is that a hypothesis can provide the best explanation of certain data. To put the matter roughly and crudely, two conditions need to be fulfilled. It needs to be the case that the data would be expected if the hypothesis were true. And it also needs to be the case that the data would not be expected if the hypothesis were not true. So let us now apply those conditions.

We have already seen that the first condition is fulfilled. The sanctity of human life is *entailed* by the theistic picture. So if the theistic picture were true, then we would not be at all surprised to find that we have been granted an intuitive sense of the value of each human life; or that people who tap the resources described by that picture are motivated to reach out in care to otherwise uncared-for individuals; or that we regard the committed care that we there observe as entirely fitting.

And in fact, we do see the theistic picture informing and motivating countless people, like Mother Teresa, to provide that care. Of course, those people do not believe the theistic picture on the ground that it provides the best explanation of their intuitions about the value of each individual. They believe their picture on many other independent grounds – the historical, theological, philosophical and personal grounds for believing the Judaeo-Christian narrative to be true. But because they believe this narrative, they accept the entailed doctrine of the sanctity of human life. Mother Teresa and the other carers would claim that the theistic narrative enables them to recognise each damaged human life, however grossly deformed, at least to some extent as God regards it, as the life of a precious individual for whom God has purposes beyond anything visible to us now. And they would also claim that the love which they extend to those for whom they care is a love which comes to them from God. As we saw in Chapter Three, the truth of what they claim to see, and the power of the love they claim to receive, are exactly what we would expect if the theistic picture is true.

And if that picture is true, then others of us – those of us who are not so readily moved to provide that kind of care – might nevertheless feel inspired by the example we see in Mother Teresa and like-minded carers, because their care resonates with the intuitive sense we have been granted of the sanctity of life, and so we feel that the love there on display is not misplaced and misguided, but wonderful.

So the first condition is indeed fulfilled. The data are certainly to be expected if the hypothesis is true.

What, then, of the second condition? Are we in a position to say that the data would not be expected if the hypothesis were not true?

Peter Singer certainly believes that this condition is fulfilled. He believes that Christianity is the culprit: if we can rid ourselves of Christian belief, we can then rid ourselves of the misleading intuitions concerning the sanctity of life, and we can reform the misguided conduct inspired by this false doctrine – as other cultures have managed to do. He believes that the data would disappear if we concerned ourselves with the evident, natural facts, and with our own reasonable inferences drawn from those facts. He and Glover both seek to persuade us to abandon the doctrine of the sanctity of life by directing our attention to those natural facts.

And Singer and Glover seem to be correct in insisting that the doctrine of the sanctity of life cannot be grounded in what is merely natural. In order to convince us of the value of the lives of the disabled, advocates for the disabled tend to direct our attention to the many abilities which disabled persons possess in spite of their bodily condition. But not every disabled person readily displays such abilities: some disabilities are so severe that the value of that person's life is not presented to us in that way. When we see a grossly damaged human life as precious in the same fundamental way as a normal life is precious, we cannot be seeing what is presented solely by the natural facts before us. It seems that we must be sensing a truth which transcends those natural facts.

Nor, it seems, can the behaviour of those who are motivated by the doctrine be explained in the usual naturalistic terms. *Evolutionary* processes provide the standard model for the naturalistic explanations of human features. The naturalist typically seeks to explain all our inclinations, our attitudes, our abilities, our behaviour, in terms of some account of how these features are conducive to the survival of the human species. But it would obviously be extremely difficult to provide any plausible evolutionary explanation of the love demonstrated by Mother Teresa and the others, because the individuals for whom they care are precisely *not* those whose continued existence would be conducive to the survival of the species. And for just the same reason, it would be similarly difficult to provide any evolutionary explanation of our intuition concerning the value of each damaged human life, or of the fact that we are inspired when we observe the love invested in its care.

And nor, it seems, will the behaviour of Mother Teresa and others be easily explained simply in terms of their natural inclinations to care. For these carers profess that they *depend upon* the *insight* provided by God in order to recognise the need for their work and upon the *power* provided by God in order to be moved and enabled to do that work. They claim, in other words, that their work would not arise simply from their own natural inclinations. And this claim of theirs receives support from such considerations as the following.

The theistic picture does not imply that only those who believe that picture will engage in committed care for compromised human life. As we saw in Chapter Three, that picture entails that we *all* have moral knowledge and that we can all grow in virtue, so it offers us reason not to be surprised when we see morally sensitive persons of any persuasion reaching out in compassion and selfless care to those in need. But it must be admitted that the kind of example displayed by Mother Teresa and others is unusual. As Singer stresses, it is unusual culturally and historically. And in many ways, it actually runs counter to our natural inclinations. Even though we may intuitively accept that each life has its own value, and though we may be inspired once we see before us the example presented by Mother Teresa and others, it is easy for us to *fail* to see grossly deformed human life as calling for our care, and it is certainly very easy for us to fail to be motivated to provide that care. As Glover and Singer insist, we cannot see the value of such life merely by inspecting its natural qualities. And, as I am ashamed to note, we can naturally find such damaged human life to be very off-putting, indeed repulsive. We may prefer not even to know about it, much less to engage with it. And we can be deeply disinclined to expend the effort required in its care. Thus we can be all too ready to ignore it altogether; or, if we cannot avoid considering it, to acquiesce in a dismissive attitude towards it. And so we are readily able to suppress our truthful intuition concerning the value of such life and to rationalise our decisions to withhold care.

But as we saw in Chapter Three, the theist will claim not only that we all have moral knowledge and ability, but also that in our moral deliberation and behaviour we would be foolish to try to proceed without keeping the whole truth in view, as it is described by the theistic narrative. We need the information provided by that narrative if we are to *recognise fully* what our moral duties are. And we need to appropriate the help described by that narrative if we are to be properly *moved and enabled to perform* our moral duties – for we need to call upon the transforming power of God. So says the theist. And Mother Teresa and the innumerable like-minded carers would claim that this is exactly what is going on in their work. They claim that the theistic narrative *reveals to* them the true, incalculable value of each human; and that it shows this to them with a *clarity* which cuts through our natural blindness and our rationalisations and self-deceptions – the rationalisations which enable the rest of us to ignore the needy individuals. The theistic narrative, the carers say, both requires and enables them to *see* each damaged human life as precious to God and deserving of our care. And they claim that they are *empowered* by, and with, a love which exceeds what their own natural resources can provide. They claim that they *need* to draw upon the love of God in this way. And as we watch their love at work, we are inspired precisely because we are reacting to a phenomenon which appears not to be entirely natural, and because we are lifted beyond our own natural inclinations.

Even so, might not Mother Teresa and the others just happen to be extraordinary people who find themselves with temperaments of such a kind that they feel a natural affection for the individuals for whom they care? But this is a deeply implausible suggestion. It is of course true that many of our commitments of care – in marriage, in the family, in friendship, and so on – are commitments which arise from our natural inclinations and desires and affections. But sometimes it is exactly the other way around: a felt affection might eventually *emerge* from a relationship of care which is first forged from a *commitment* made by the carer. Every dedicated nurse knows how it can in time become very difficult to say goodbye to a patient for whom she has devotedly cared, but for whom she initially felt no natural affection. Her emergent affection arises as a product of the commitment to care, not *vice versa*. And the rest of us can experience something similar even in our natural relationships. For we all find that times arrive when a willed commitment is required if our important relationships are to be maintained, because the original, merely natural affection loses its power; but the renewed commitment can produce a renewed affection. Now the care provided by Mother Teresa and others is much more plausibly explained as due to chosen commitment rather than to natural affection. They choose to reach out to grossly damaged individuals who have already been abandoned by their natural families. These are individuals for whom *their own families* feel no natural affection. Nor, typically, do the rest of us feel any natural affection for these individuals. I have already noted that we are all too easily repelled by what we see when we are forced to look at these deformed lives. But Mother Teresa and the others commit themselves to the care of these individuals because of what they *believe* – that each individual is precious to God, and deserving of our care. These carers claim that they are relying on the insight provided to them by God, and that they need to refresh this perspective continually. For they do not merely initiate their care: they *persist* in it as a settled commitment. And there is nothing easy about this. Again, every dedicated nurse can testify to how difficult it is to persevere in the relentless grind of the care for the profoundly disabled or demented. But Mother Teresa and the others press on in their committed care, with regularly renewed motivation. Indeed, they do so not merely with the kind of affection the rest of us might display in our ordinary relationships, but with evident and persistent love – and indeed, with joy. And they claim, once again, that all of this comes from God. In claiming this, they are of course taking for granted that they would not *otherwise* be able to do their work as they do. They are claiming that without their being constantly refreshed in the theistic perspective, and without their being constantly renewed in God's love, their work would not go on. They are implying, in other words, that their loving care would not occur *unless* God were in the business of informing and transforming and empowering them. And this certainly seems to accord with our own observations about how extraordinary their love is. They do seem to be maintaining an unnatural perspective, and to be drawing upon an unnatural fuel. Yet their work is utterly realistic. They are clearly not operating under the influence of some mind-altering drug or artificial stimulant. Each new day, their sleeves are rolled up in thoroughly clear-sighted, earthy devotion to the care of the neediest.

These considerations certainly suggest, then, that the care provided by Mother Teresa and others *depends upon* the truth of the theistic picture – that if that picture were not true, then such care would not be on display.

So there does seem to be good reason to conclude that the data are not to be expected if the theistic picture is not true, and therefore that the second condition is fulfilled.

Both conditions, then, appear to be fulfilled. The loving care which is displayed by Mother Teresa and countless like-minded carers, and the fact that their care squares with the intuitive but unnatural sense that we possess of the value of each human life, and the fact that such care inspires us beyond our own natural inclinations, are all to be expected if the theistic picture is true, but not to be expected if the theistic picture is not true. And this strongly suggests that the theistic picture does indeed provide the best explanation of those data. In which case, of course, we have here real evidence of the truth of the theistic picture. And if this picture is true, then we too can be empowered to care in the way in which those countless others have been empowered.

It seems to me very interesting that our ethical thinking is in this way leading us into metaphysics – the subject concerned with questions about the fundamental nature of reality, the existence of God, the nature and significance of the human person, the meaning of life, and so on. Those are exciting questions; but their discussion takes us, I'm afraid, beyond the scope of this book.

But what is certainly not beyond the scope of this book is the fact that we need to take very seriously a particularly stark contrast which we have now observed. We have seen two different approaches to the question of disability and selective infanticide, which have proceeded from two very different views of the significance of human life and death. And those views have their own very different sets of implications for our understanding of the duty of care at the heart of the caring professions. To whom do we have such a duty? And just what sort of duty is it?

On the one hand, there is the view that some human lives are disposable and replaceable; that destroying a human life might be no more morally serious than our choosing not to conceive a child; that we may withhold our care from, and indeed destroy, unwanted lives; that whether an individual is to be cared for, and indeed allowed to continue to exist, can be determined by what *we* think about whether his or her life would be worthwhile; and so on.

On the other hand, there is the view that *each* human life is precious, however damaged or disabled or deranged or unwanted it may be; and that it deserves our committed, supportive care.

Which kind of carer shall we seek to be?

Notes

1 See, for instance, Julian Savulescu, "Procreative Beneficence: Why We Should Select the Best Children", *Bioethics*, 15 (October 2001), pp. 414–26.
2 Stella Young, "We are more than the sum of our genes", on *Ramp Up*, the ABC Blog on Disability, 9th October 2012, at www.abc.net.au/rampup/articles/2012/10/09/3606293.htm
3 Rosalind Hursthouse offers a penetrating discussion of how our talk about disability can be callously insensitive to the obvious value of the lives of many disabled people, and how those people themselves, and their parents, can understandably find such talk "enraging, insulting, hurtful, devastating – and threatening". See her *Beginning Lives* (Blackwell/Open University, Oxford, 1987), pp. 213–6.
4 Ronald Munson, *Intervention and Reflection: Basic Issues in Medical Ethics*, Eighth Edition (Thomson, Belmont, 2008), p. 302.
5 Hursthouse provides a very helpful review of this range of considerations, and of the insight we can gain by thinking about them in terms of the requirements of the virtues. See her book *Beginning Lives*, *op. cit.*, and her article "Virtue Theory and Abortion", *Philosophy and Public Affairs*, Vol. 20, No. 3, pp. 223–46.
6 For example, Michael Tooley, "Abortion and Infanticide", *Philosophy & Public Affairs*, Vol. 2, No. 1, pp. 37–65 (1972); Jonathan Glover, *Causing Death and Saving Lives* (Penguin, Harmondsworth, 1977); Peter Singer, *Practical Ethics* (Cambridge University Press, Cambridge, 1979).
7 This, at least, is the "official" position within general Western medical ethics. But medical practice can be murkier. The *Arthur* case in the United Kingdom in 1981 demonstrated considerable medical professional support for Dr Arthur's withholding of life-preserving treatment from a Down's syndrome baby not wanted

by its parents. And Peter Singer cites evidence that many other disabled infants are allowed to die. *Op. cit.*, pp. 147–9. (Singer regards this as a step in the right direction. But he believes that medical practice ought to go further and allow the active killing of such babies.)

8 I do not know enough about Mother Teresa to be able to offer a detailed evaluation of her work. (Aspects of her work have been criticised by some, and I am not in a position to assess those criticisms in proper detail.) But I refer to her here as an example of what she is known and admired for throughout the world – as an example of selfless dedication to the care of the neediest, including abandoned babies.

9 Jonathan Glover, *op. cit.* Chapters 3, 8 and 12 are the parts of the book most relevant to our discussion here.

10 Peter Singer, *op. cit.* Singer was a student at Glover's seminars at Oxford. Singer discusses Glover's influence upon his own work in Benoit Basse, "An Interview with Peter Singer on Jonathan Glover and the Ethics of Killing", *Canadian Journal of Bioethics*, Vol. 2, No. 1, 2019, pp. 77–83. There has been a great deal of further discussion and development of their ideas since Glover and Singer first presented them in their highly influential early writings. But I will not try to engage with any of that here. As is my strategy throughout this book, I am not trying to provide a scholarly overview of the topic, but rather to expose and discuss the *basic questions* that I believe the caring professions need to face. Glover's and Singer's landmark texts are ideal for this purpose.

11 Glover, *op. cit.*, p. 161.

12 *Ibid.*, pp. 163–4. (Glover's emphasis.)

13 Michael Tooley (*op. cit.*) and Peter Singer (*op. cit.*) both seek to draw far-reaching moral implications from the fact that the infant cannot *now* have a preference to continue to live – as an ongoing, distinct entity – rather than to die. Tooley argues that this entails that the infant does not have a right to life. Singer argues that this shows that the infant has no preference that needs to be considered by the preference utilitarian. And both of them appeal to this fact as part of their reason for claiming that the infant is not a *person*. It seems to me that each of their positions is vulnerable to what I have said in response to Glover's dismissal of autonomy.

14 Singer, *op. cit.*, p. 100. Singer and Glover are here talking about sentient life, not the life of self-conscious, autonomous individuals. (And thus they take themselves to be talking about human babies.)

15 Glover, *op. cit.*, p. 159.

16 *Ibid.*, p. 159.

17 *Ibid.*, p. 159 (Glover's emphasis).

18 *Ibid.*, p. 159.

19 *Ibid.*, p. 40.

20 *Ibid.*, pp. 162–3.

21 *Ibid.*

22 *Ibid.*, pp. 45–50.

23 *Ibid.*, p. 47.

24 Singer, *op. cit.*, pp. 77–8, 125.

25 See note 8, above.

Index

For Product Safety Concerns and Information please contact our EU representative GPSR@taylorandfrancis.com
Taylor & Francis Verlag GmbH, Kaufingerstraße 24, 80331 München, Germany

www.ingramcontent.com/pod-product-compliance
Lightning Source LLC
LaVergne TN
LVHW021125300926
849160LV00010B/865
9781032009582